IMAGES
of America

J. C. BLAIR
MEMORIAL HOSPITAL

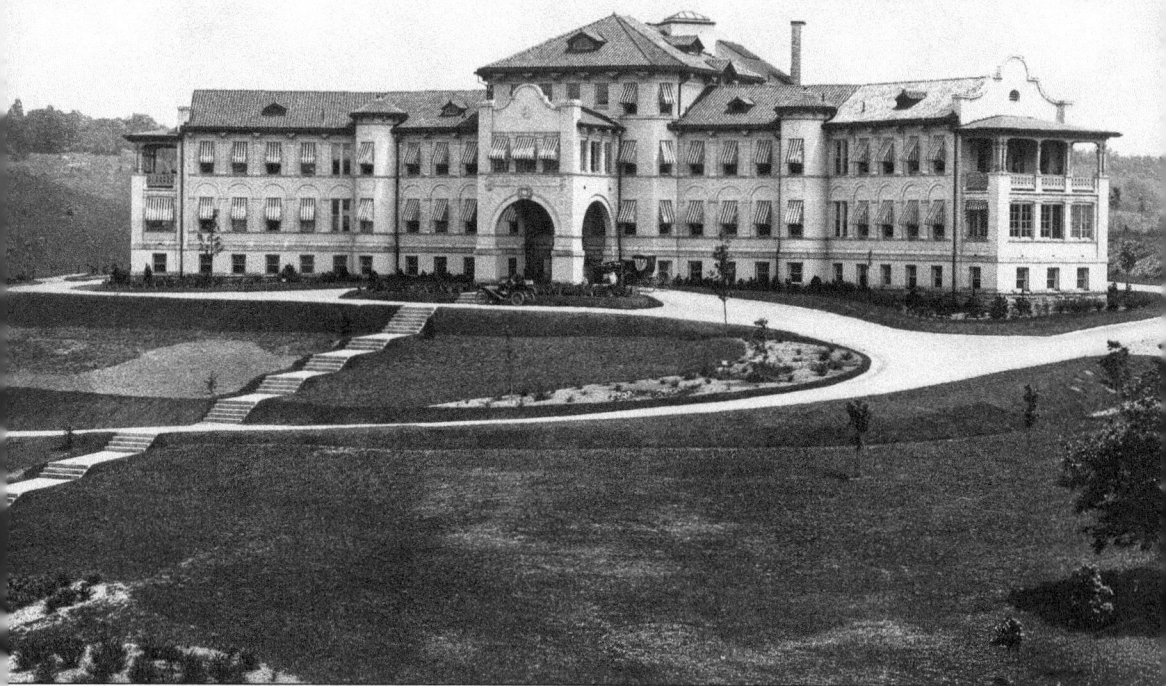

With gaily striped awnings shading every window, J. C. Blair Memorial Hospital looks in this historic image as much like a first-class resort hotel as the hospital it actually is. Perched atop a hill overlooking the town of Huntingdon, Pennsylvania, the hospital embodied the dream of its donor, Kate Fisher Blair, and her late husband, who together conceived the idea of this healing institution to serve the community they loved. (Courtesy of Huntingdon County Historical Society.)

ON THE COVER: This private patient in the new J. C. Blair Memorial Hospital appears to lack nothing that could speed her recovery. Two nurses stand ready to fluff her pillows and pour her tea. A vase of roses brightens her well-appointed room, complete with a handsome brass bed. Her shoulders are warmed by the bed jacket she wears, and a chenille robe awaits at the foot of the bed should she need it. (Courtesy of Huntingdon County Historical Society.)

IMAGES
of America

J. C. Blair
Memorial Hospital

Nancy Swigart Shedd
and Alberta Haught Goshorn

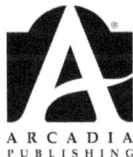

ARCADIA
PUBLISHING

Published by Arcadia Publishing
Charleston SC, Chicago IL, Portsmouth NH, San Francisco CA

Library of Congress Control Number: 2009942365

For all general information contact Arcadia Publishing at:
Telephone 843-853-2070
Fax 843-853-0044
E-mail sales@arcadiapublishing.com
For customer service and orders:
Toll-Free 1-888-313-2665

Visit us on the Internet at www.arcadiapublishing.com

To the bold thinkers and doers of J. C. Blair Memorial Hospital's early years, who dreamed of what could be—and worked to achieve that dream

CONTENTS

ACKNOWLEDGMENTS

A hospital is a community institution in which we all have a stake; therefore, it is heartening that the community has participated so generously in producing this book. Our thanks to all.

Major contributions have come from the Huntingdon County Historical Society, which holds the archives that tell the history of J. C. Blair Memorial Hospital. Executive director Jennifer Stahl and her assistant, Kelley Kroecker, worked closely with us. News editor Polly McMullin and writer Becky Weikert of *The Daily News* responded willingly to every request we made. Blair Hospital's Chris Gildea and Blair Foundation's Marsha Hartman cooperated fully, answering many questions. And words fail us when trying to express what a pleasure it has been to work with Fred Lang, who scanned all the images for the book. The project truly would not have been possible without his expertise and unfailing good humor.

We are grateful for research assistance from Brady Smith, an expert at searching *The Daily News* online; Pat Beck, who mined *The Daily News* morgue for doctors; Alice Heine, who answered many questions; and Ray Brooks, who found obituaries of key figures. Longtime hospital board president John Kunz shared his hospital archive; Bob Cree found Virginia Filiatreault; Robert Vaughn knew where the surviving Faulkner triplets were; Vicky Huggler located lost photographs and made identifications; Vickie Russell helped with the Beck Collection; Elizabeth Goodman answered Mount Union questions; Sam Miller found Hartslog Museum material; Roy Stevens answered Three Springs/Saltillo requests; Jon Baughman, Ron Morgan, and Adam Watson gave Broad Top area help.

Virginia Bollman Filiatreault is one of less than a handful of surviving graduates of Blair's Nurses Training School, which closed with her class of 1940. We are delighted that Virginia wrote down her memories of nursing school and military service for us.

Images in this book not otherwise credited are from the collections of the Huntingdon County Historical Society. People who shared photographs are credited where those images appear. The late Dr. Robert Beck's collection of doctor photographs is credited BC. Photographs from *The Daily News* are credited TDN.

INTRODUCTION

When Kate Fisher Blair announced on January 1, 1909, that she intended to give a hospital to the community in memory of her husband, J. C. Blair, it was a defining moment in the history of Huntingdon and the county that surrounds it. A community with a hospital becomes essentially different from a community without one, and that difference goes beyond the obvious fact that the area benefits from its proximity to the medical care available only in a hospital setting. In addition, it enjoys not only the institution's offer of employment to a broad segment of its citizens, but also the benefit of having those associated with the hospital live within its boundaries, where their participation in other community institutions—churches, schools, and charitable organizations, not to mention its economy—enhances the entire area's quality of life.

J. C. Blair Memorial Hospital was a fitting memorial to a man whose ideas and actions had benefited his community in so many ways during his life. The successful business he built from scratch grew rapidly and offered steady employment to hundreds of his fellow citizens. The innovative thinking, which propelled the development of the products he manufactured, led him to adopt many business practices that were advanced for the time. He encouraged his employees' interests and talents by sponsoring ball teams and an orchestra. He recognized those with special promise, including women, promoting them to positions of responsibility and helping them to develop their abilities to the fullest.

J. C. Blair Memorial Hospital's birth occurred at a time when reform movements were underway in hospitals, medical schools, and nursing schools. Historically, hospitals cared for the destitute and housed the homeless and chronically ill. There were no trained nurses to care for the sick and dying that populated the hospitals of the 18th and early 19th centuries, as the country's first nursing schools were not founded until 1873. Patients who were able to work did what tasks they could, often in the most slovenly and unsanitary fashion.

But, over time, advances in medical knowledge and the reform efforts of Florence Nightingale and others resulted in better education of doctors and of professionally trained nurses. Together they combined to raise standards and create a new image of what a hospital might be.

Beginning in the late 1880s, communities desiring to bring the services of these professionals to their residents encouraged the founding of hospitals in towns that previously had no local institutions dedicated to providing medical care. J. C. Blair Memorial Hospital came to life in this context, as a community hospital dedicated to serving the needs of the residents of Huntingdon County.

To carry the idea of a hospital forward and make it a reality, Kate Fisher Blair named 13 men to a commission charged with developing the project. They were responsible for making the decisions that brought the hospital into being and for managing its finances. The commission was the forerunner of the institution's board of trustees. Through the years, the board has been composed of community members, who have contributed the knowledge and expertise gained in their particular realms of experience—in business, banking, law, medicine, and other careers—to the operation and management of the hospital. These leaders have guided the expansion of the physical plant and of the medical services offered and have established the policies that govern the operation of the institution they oversee.

Within a few months of its opening in 1911, Blair Hospital welcomed five young women to its Nurses Training School, thus embarking on a 30-year period of activity in which 186 registered nurses would be graduated. Doctors on the hospital staff instructed these aspiring nurses in their three-year course of study—a considerable commitment of their time and attention, on top of running their individual practices. The dedication of this early corps of doctors, to the hospital and the nursing school, laid the foundation upon which the institution has built during the following century.

Dedication is a word that can be applied as well to the women who chartered the Ladies' Auxiliary in 1913. Like the doctors, they devoted uncounted hours of their time—providing amenities for patients and student nurses; fund-raising to purchase needed equipment; making and mending countless towels, nightgowns, and sheets; and covering the annual deficit in the hospital's early years. Their sustained support has been more essential than is often recognized in enabling the hospital to reach its 100th anniversary.

For 35 years, J. C. Blair Memorial Hospital's original building adapted to the increased demands the growing community placed on it. But, in 1946, the trustees could see that expansion of the physical plant was essential. They hired the hospital's first professional administrator to lead a major fund-raising campaign for the construction of a building that would more than double the institution's capacity and would modernize the entire facility. Again, as at the hospital's beginning, the board was farsighted enough to construct a building with room for future expansion and adaptation. With additions and modifications, it remains the center of the institution's present complex.

The hospital's original building did not survive to celebrate its 100th birthday. It was doomed, in part, by its solid-masonry fireproof construction, which prevented reconfiguration of its interior spaces and made updating its wiring, plumbing, and heating systems difficult and expensive. There is no doubt that the building was iconic; it created lasting images in the minds of those to whom it was a familiar sight for so many years. Proof of that resides in the entrance created for the 1950 building after the 1911 building was demolished, an entrance that, in effect, recreates the original porte cochere and echoes the profile of the old building's curvilinear gables.

The celebration of a 100th anniversary calls for a look back and provokes a gasp of astonishment at how much has changed. It is a huge jump from horse-drawn ambulances to medevac helicopters. Fortunately, change typically comes in manageable steps, not in jumps. And J. C. Blair Memorial Hospital has proven itself capable of taking those steps—with the cooperation and support of its many constituencies—in order to end its first century well-prepared to embark upon its second.

One

THE BLAIRS

When John Chalmers Blair died on June 23, 1897, he was just 49 years old. In a life cut prematurely short, he had achieved the greatest entrepreneurial success ever attained by a Huntingdon County native son.

In a little store on Huntingdon's "Diamond," Blair began his career selling books, novelties, wallpaper, and sewing machines. On a press in the back room, he printed Sunday school reward cards, given to children in recognition of perfect attendance or the memorization of Bible verses.

One day in the late 1870s, Blair watched his friend David Emmert, an art teacher at the Brethren Normal College, cut and staple together sheets of blank paper on which to draw or write. A light bulb went on in J. C.'s mind. Soon his wife, Kate, was cooking up batches of glue in their kitchen, and he was experimenting with how to make a paper tablet that could be produced commercially.

The tablet was the humble item upon which Blair's great success was founded. His genius was in attaching to the tablets brightly colored and well-designed covers that made them sell like the proverbial hotcakes.

The rapid expansion of Blair's business can be tracked by the size of the buildings that contained it: from the little store on the "Diamond" to the mammoth eight-story building that still dominates Huntingdon's skyline. By the time it was built, Blair's tablets were selling all over the world, and the manufacturing stationers trade association had recognized him as the inventor of the paper tablet.

Guiding the business required Blair's close attention, but not to the exclusion of other concerns on which he expended the same devotion and innovative thinking. He served on the borough council and as chief burgess, donated athletic fields, funded street paving, established company baseball teams and an orchestra, and proposed erecting a memorial Standing Stone.

Clearly J. C. Blair's honored place in area history rests upon the broad foundation laid during his lifetime and enhanced by Kate Blair's continuing contributions to the community in his memory.

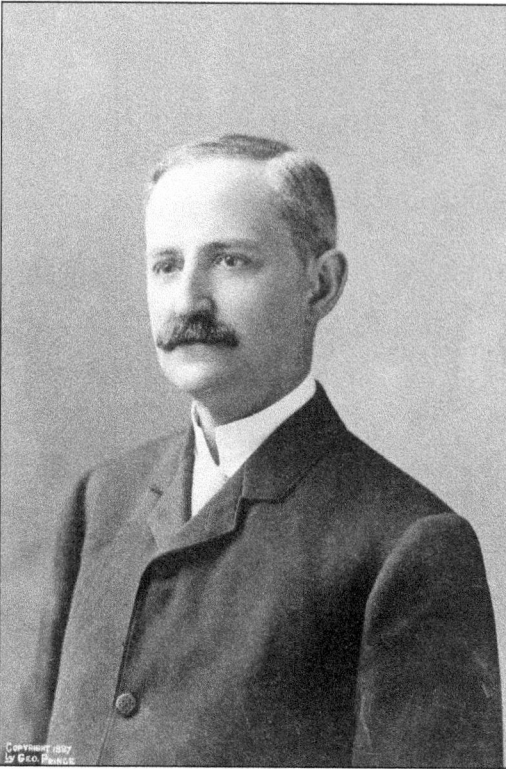

J. C. Blair was born August 14, 1847, near Shade Gap, to Brice X. and Amanda Blair. On a visit to "the Shades" six months later, David Blair admired his young nephew and pronounced him "a remarkably healthy heavy boy." David judged the young one to be "as heavy as two turkies." "They call him John Chalmers," he wrote in a letter to his wife.

The inventiveness of 19th-century typography and design are displayed to advantage in this invitation to the wedding of Kate Fisher and J. C. Blair. Graphic design and color lithography became the stock in trade of Blair's business success.

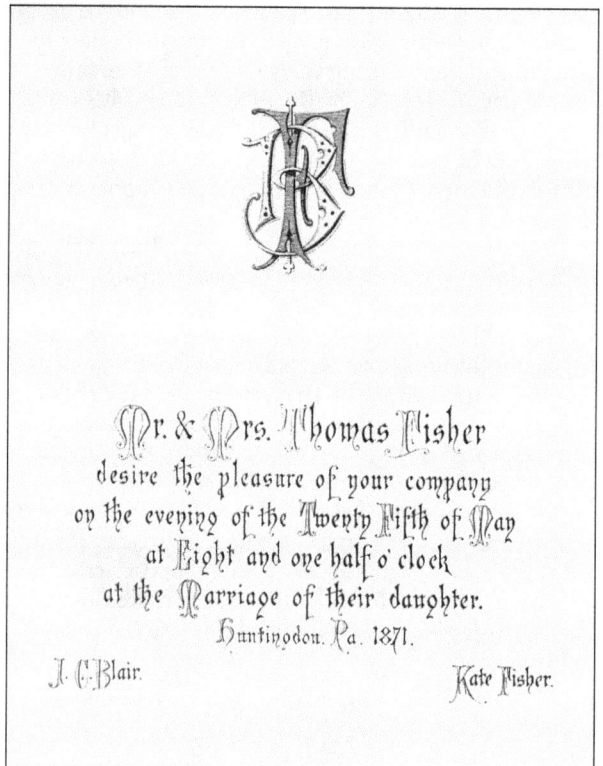

Mr. & Mrs. Thomas Fisher
desire the pleasure of your company
on the evening of the Twenty Fifth of May
at Eight and one half o' clock
at the Marriage of their daughter.
Huntingdon. Pa. 1871.

J. C. Blair.   Kate Fisher.

Next to the youngest of the 10 children of Thomas and Rebecca Jackson Fisher was Kate, who would become Mrs. J. C. Blair. Kate grew up in the house her father built at 222 Penn Street and was connected through her aunts, uncles, cousins, and siblings with many of Huntingdon's old families. Thomas Fisher clerked for various merchants early in his career and, in 1855, established the highly successful Huntingdon Mills at Seventh and Penn Streets.

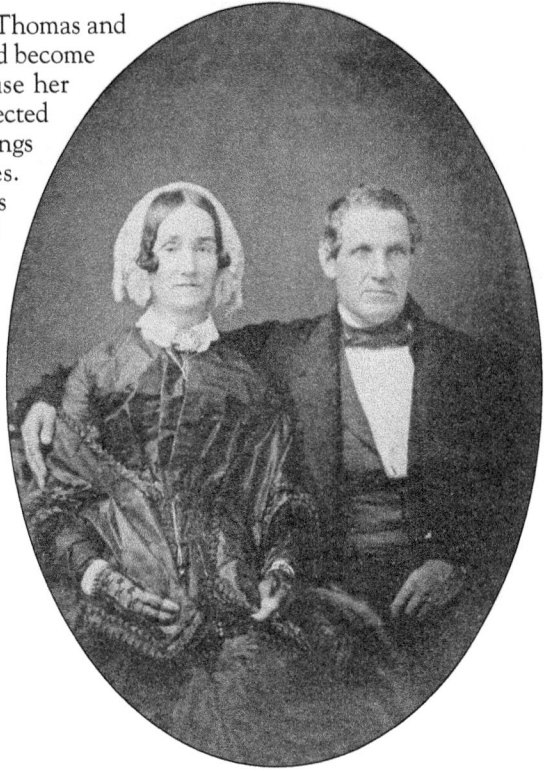

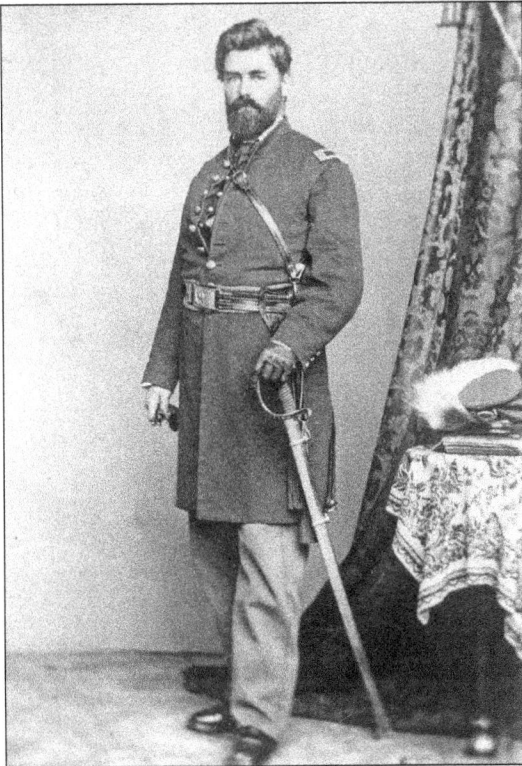

J. C. Blair revered his father's military service during the Civil War. Captain of Company I, 149th Regiment, Pennsylvania Volunteers, Brice X. Blair lost his left arm July 1, 1863, at Gettysburg. After the war, he was appointed postmaster at Huntingdon by President Grant and moved his family to a house on Fourth Street.

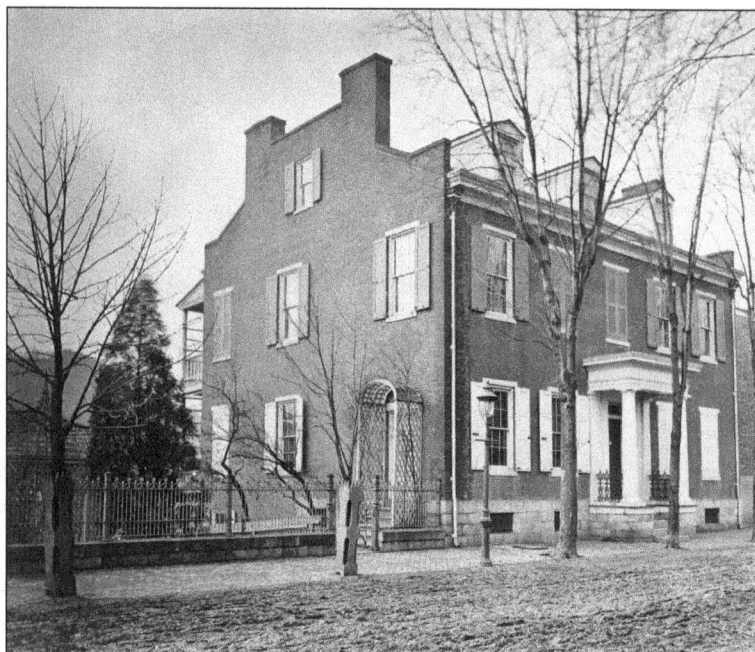

The fine house Thomas Fisher built in 1850 for his large family was located just across the street from the county's 1842 Greek Revival courthouse. The generously proportioned house offered four useable stories, from a basement kitchen to finished bedrooms in the attic story. The four chimneys indicate a working fireplace in almost every room.

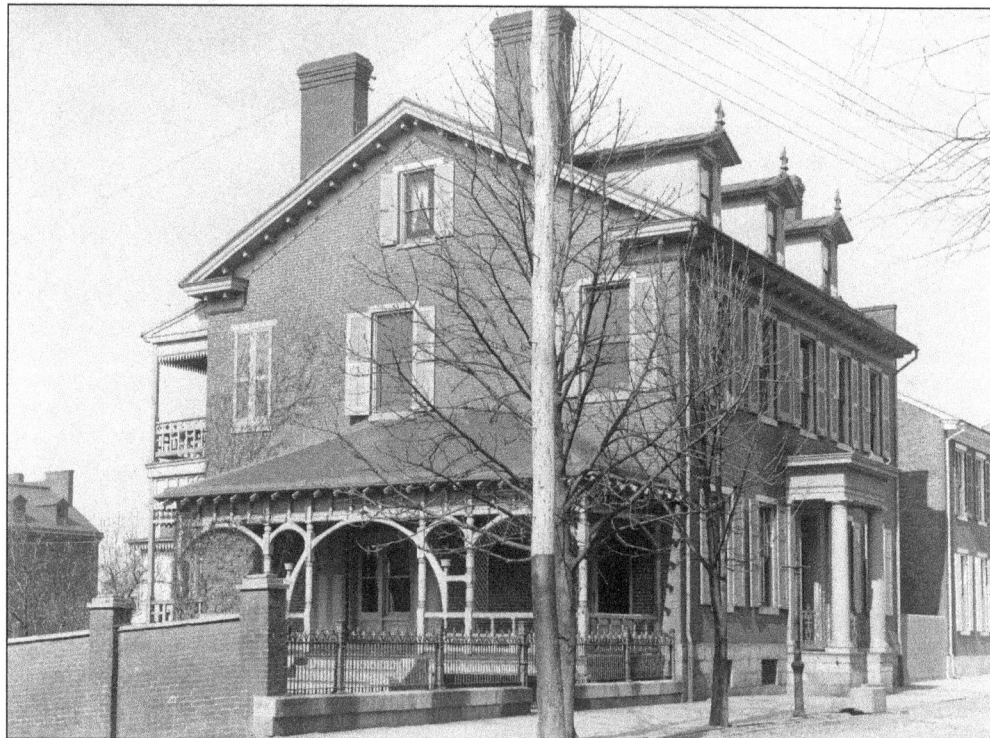

After their father's death in 1884, Kate Blair and her unmarried sister, Belle, bought the family home, where they and Kate's husband, J. C. Blair, lived. It was not long before J. C. initiated a thorough update, adding electric lights, a furnace, and other modern conveniences. In addition to the stylistic changes visible in the photograph, note the new electric pole and the absence of the gas streetlight.

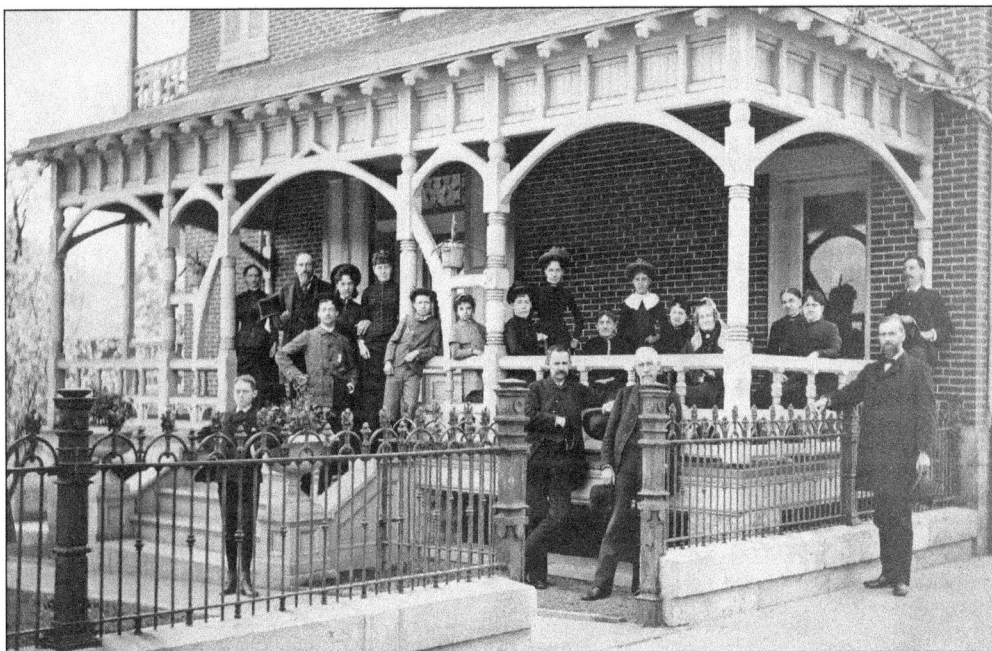

This large family group gathered on the side porch of Blair's residence is unidentified, except for the Baileys, father and son—John M. outside the fence and his son, Thomas Fisher Bailey, named for his grandfather, standing at the bottom of the steps. The dark-haired man with his hand inside his coat is J. C. Blair. Blair's and Bailey's wives, Kate and Letitia, were sisters.

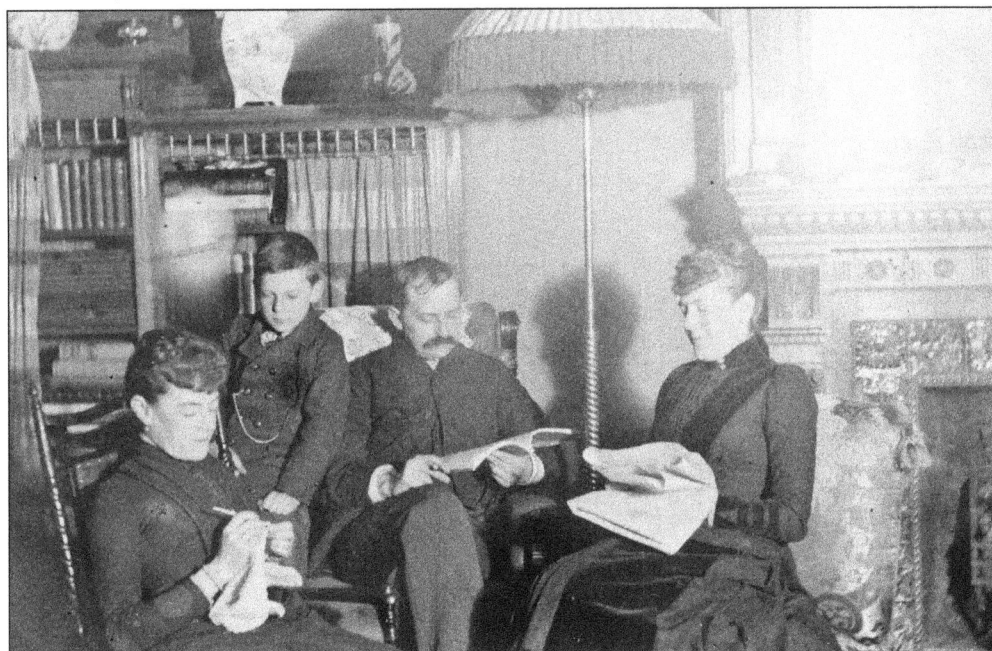

J. C. Blair's improvements to his wife's family home, which was now theirs, included interior updates in addition to the extensive changes made to the exterior. The newly available electricity lighted the large lamp that illuminated J. C. and Kate's reading and Belle's crocheting. The boy on J. C.'s right is his nephew, son of his only sibling, Cordelia Blair Jaekel.

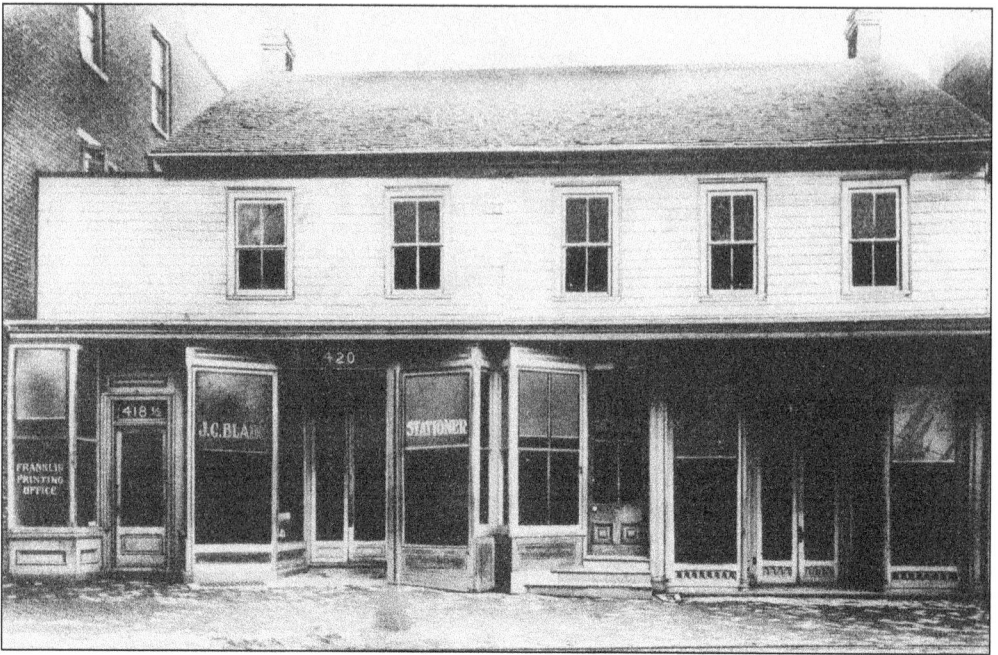

Blair went into business in this small frame store building at 420 Penn Street around 1869. Offering products as diverse as wallpaper, jewelry, and sewing machines, he struggled early in his career to find his niche. To his friend, David Emmert, he confided his aspirations: "I would like to strike a line of goods which I could manufacture in quantity."

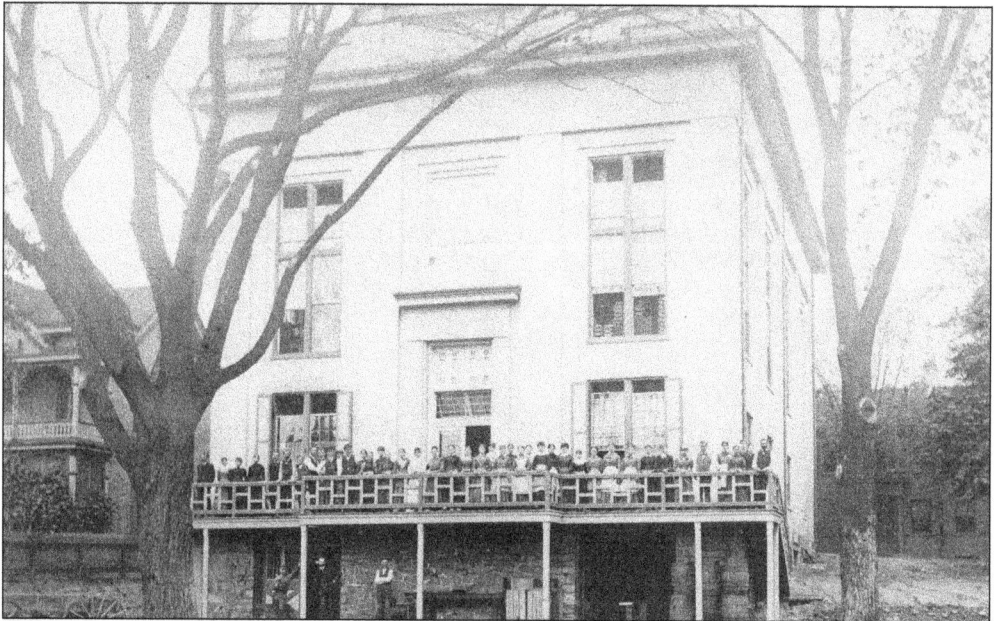

Before Blair left the little frame store, he had indeed struck on the line he could manufacture in quantity: the paper tablet. In 1881, he converted the old Presbyterian church to use as a factory, and soon, as Emmert put it, Blair's employees were "taking in hundreds of pounds of paper at the back door and sending out thousands of tablets at the front, to the amazement of the skeptical citizens of the town."

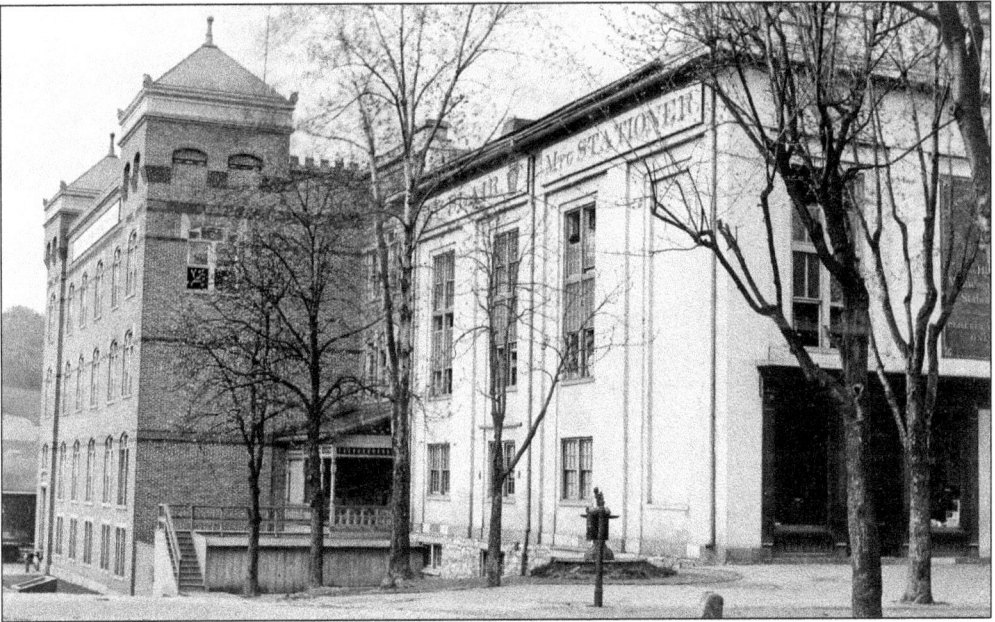

The success of Blair's line of goods was swift, and by 1884, he was building a four-story brick factory close to the railroad tracks that ran behind his manufacturing facilities. The railroad was essential to his business, bringing in the paper used in making his tablets and carrying the finished products to markets all over the country and to ports from which they were shipped all over the world.

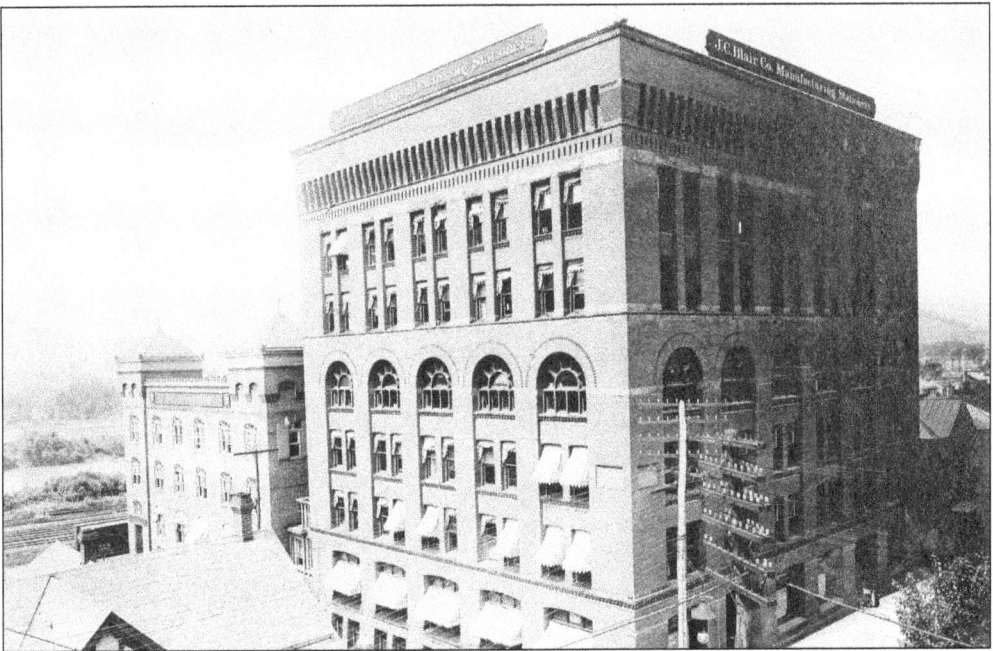

In less than five years, Blair's company required even greater expansion. Architect Frederick Olds designed a mammoth building, modeled on the renowned and much copied warehouse H. H. Richardson had built in Chicago for Marshall Field. When completed, the Blair Building was the tallest structure between Philadelphia and Pittsburgh.

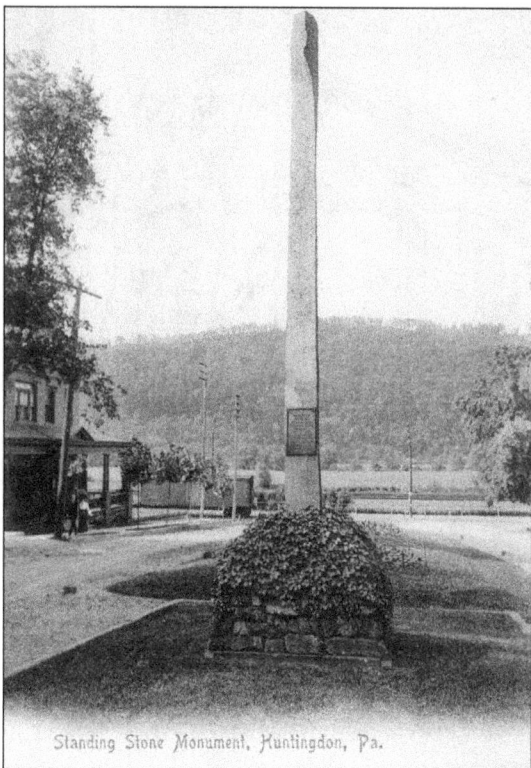

Standing Stone Monument, Huntingdon, Pa.

J. C. Blair suggested that during Huntingdon Borough's centennial in 1896, a stone monument be erected to commemorate the Indian monolith that gave the name "Standing Stone" to the area, before it was Huntingdon. Eighteenth-century travelers and settlers gave the name to nearby geographical features, now called simply Stone Creek, Stone Creek Ridge, and Stone Creek Valley.

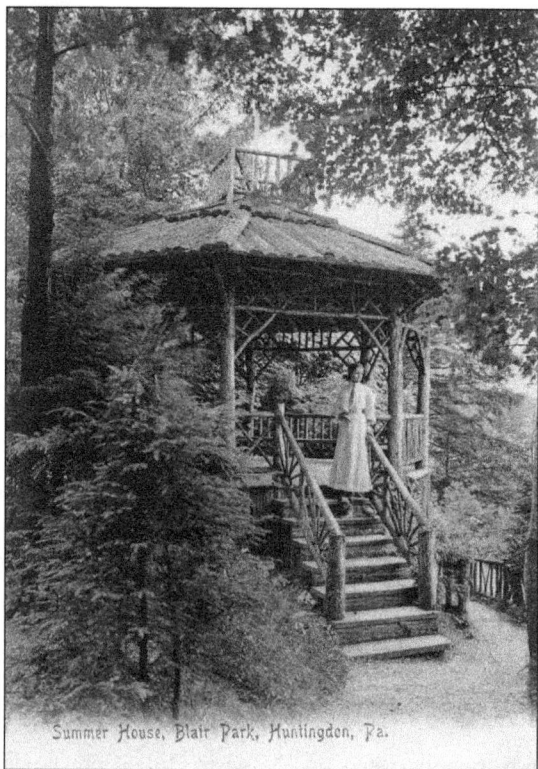

Summer House, Blair Park, Huntingdon, Pa.

Blair Park, on Huntingdon's eastern border, was laid out as a classic late-19th/early 20th-century park for strolling and driving—carriages, that is. Extending a mile or more up the creek, the park featured two rustic pavilions, railings, and a bridge. Kate Blair added this land to the athletic fields her husband had given to the borough before his death.

Two

BEGINNINGS

On New Year's Day, 1909, Kate Fisher Blair addressed a letter to Oscar H. Irwin, informing him of her intention to fund the construction of a hospital as a memorial to her late husband, J. C. Blair. She named an 11-member commission charged with overseeing all the details that accompany a major project of this kind.

Named by Kate Blair to the commission were I. Harvey Brumbaugh, president, Juniata College; C. H. Miller, president, C. H. Miller Hardware Company; Dr. Henry Clay Chisolm, physician; Harry W. Koch, vice president, J. C. Blair Company; Dr. William M. Sears, physician; Thomas F. Bailey, attorney and Kate Blair's nephew; Rev. R. P. Daubenspeck, Presbyterian minister; Samuel A. Hamilton, Pennsylvania Railroad freight agent; E. M. C. Africa, president, J. C. Blair Company; Clare M. Taylor, secretary, J. C. Blair Company; and Oscar H. Irwin, cashier, First National Bank of Huntingdon.

By February, Kate Blair had presented a check for $50,000, for the purchase of a site and for erecting and partially equipping the building. A second check in the same amount provided the beginning of an endowment. The commission had by this time selected a site known as Gernert Hill and was preparing to hold a competition to select an architect. And Kate Blair had named two additional men to the commission: Dr. Howard C. Frontz, physician; and J. Murray Africa, civil engineer.

The commission members divided themselves into eastern and western divisions for the purpose of examining existing hospitals of a size suitable for Huntingdon. When these studies were completed, specifications were drawn up and architects were invited to compete in proposing a design for the site and the building.

Three proposals were received, and Edward M. Tilton of New York City, architect of the Carnegie Library and the Stone Church of the Brethren, on the Juniata College campus, was chosen to take the project forward.

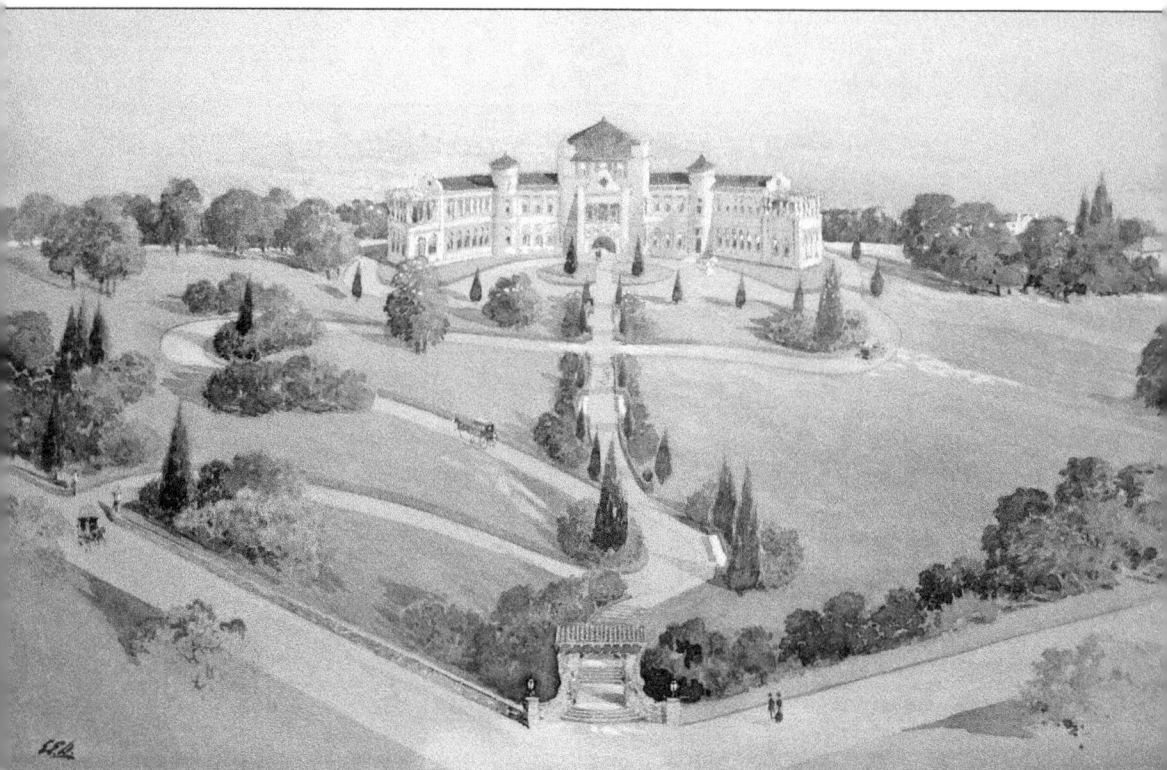

This watercolor rendering of the design that architect Edward L. Tilton proposed to the Hospital Commission persuaded them to choose his plan over those submitted by other participants in the competition for an architect. Tilton was awarded the first prize of $100; Edwin F. Bertolett, Philadelphia, $75; and Huntingdon native son Walter R. Myton, Johnstown, $50. Tilton designed more than 100 libraries during his 42-year career, many of them Carnegie libraries. Most were in classical and Beaux-Arts styles—totally unlike the Mission Revival style in which he designed the J. C. Blair Memorial Hospital. Situated on an elevated site and approached by a winding drive through landscaped grounds, the building could be a resort hotel rather than a hospital. Its design bespeaks the period's emphasis on elevation, fresh air, and sunshine as elements important to the healing of patients' bodily ills.

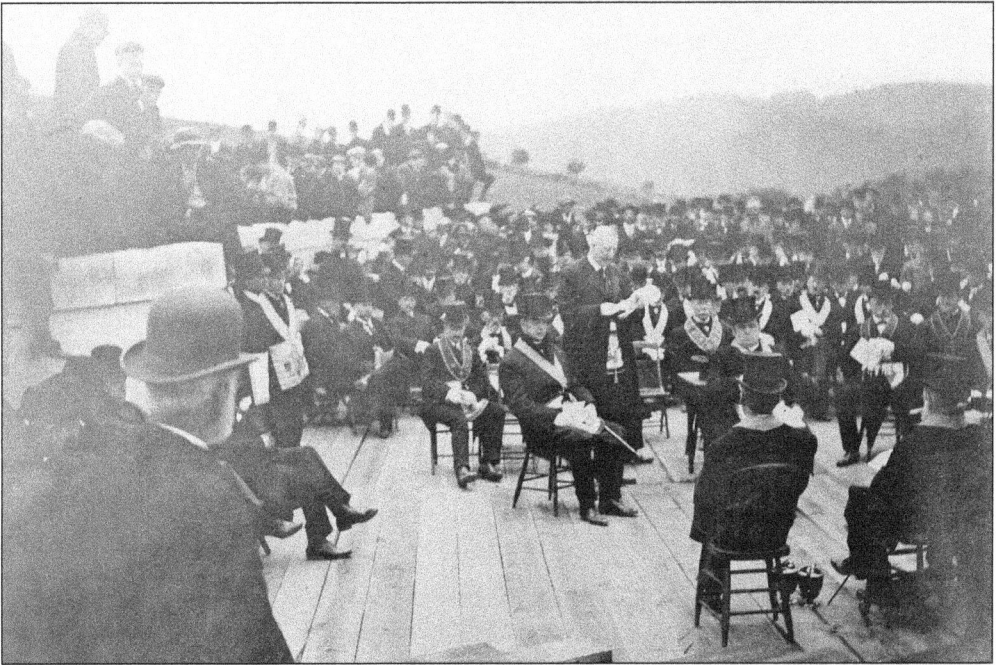

Masonic participation in cornerstone ceremonies was common in this time period. When the foundation was almost complete and a cornerstone had been prepared, it was laid with grand Masonic ceremonies on May 31, 1910. Within the cornerstone was a box, fabricated by local tinner William Hassenpflue, in which were deposited eight different Huntingdon County newspapers and other mementoes of the day.

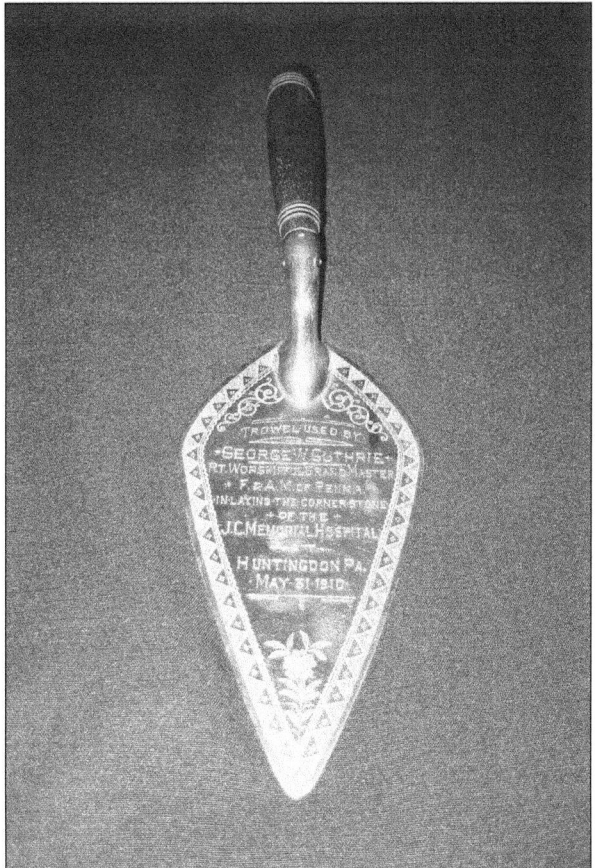

George W. Guthrie, the Right Worshipful Grand Master of Pennsylvania Masons, used this trowel to lay the cornerstone of the J. C. Blair Memorial Hospital. E. B. "Sonny" Heine Jr. found it in a building where the Masons had met for years and gave it to the hospital. The omission of the word "Blair" in the engraving was undoubtedly a serious error, which there was not time to correct. (Photograph by Linda Cutshall.)

19

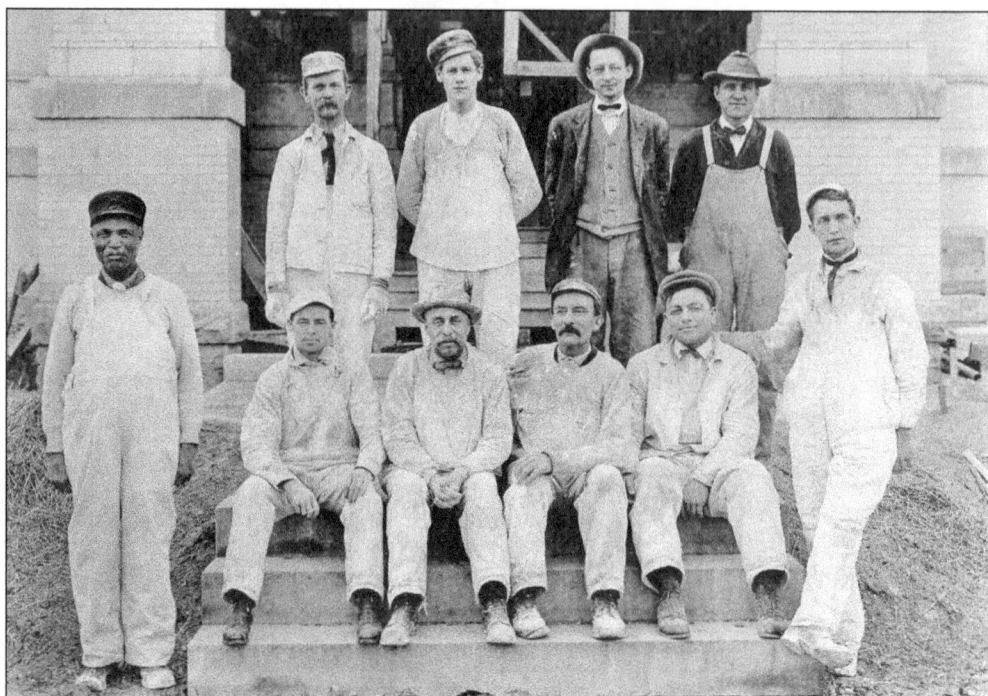

The porte cochere over the main entrance forms the background against which these workmen posed for the photographer. Their white work clothes suggest they are plasterers or painters, and the two men wearing felt hats, in the back row, are probably the crew foremen. (Courtesy of Craig Jackson.)

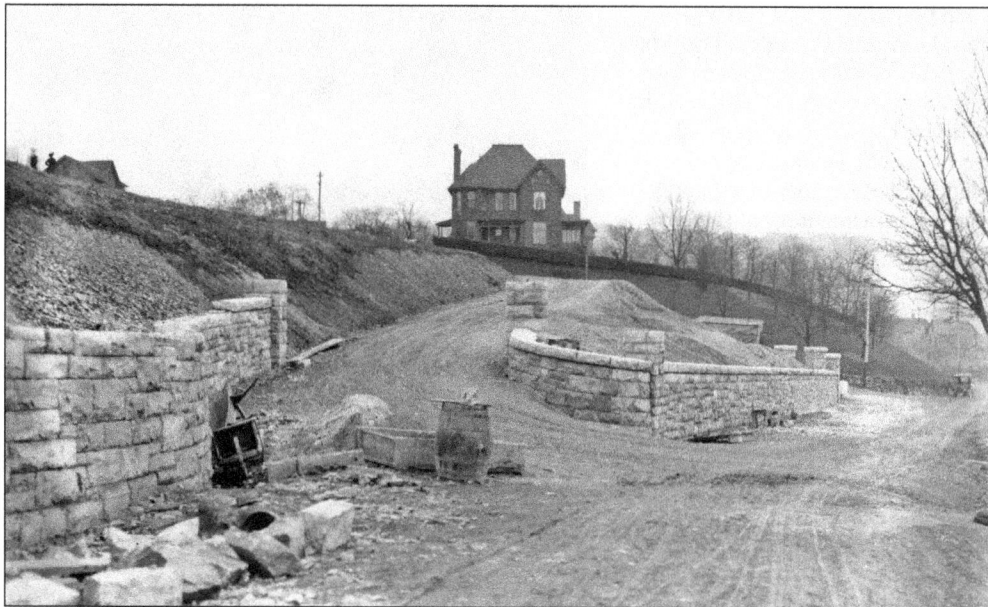

Huntingdon stonemason John Henry Gerlach was the foreman in charge of building the stone retaining wall along Warm Springs Avenue and the entrance to the winding driveway. A local newspaper reported that Gerlach's work was also exhibited in the wall surrounding the William Smith School. John D. Dorris's fine mansion looms up in the background.

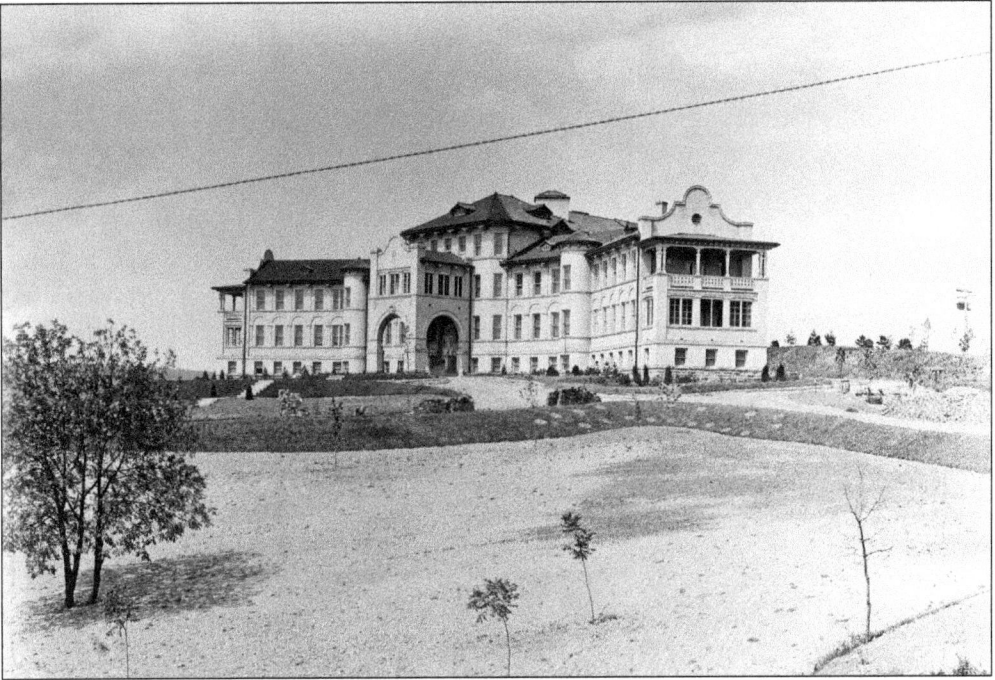

Construction of the hospital is complete in this image, which also shows that landscaping of the site has begun. Small trees and shrubs are in place, and the area in the foreground has been harrowed, ready for seeding.

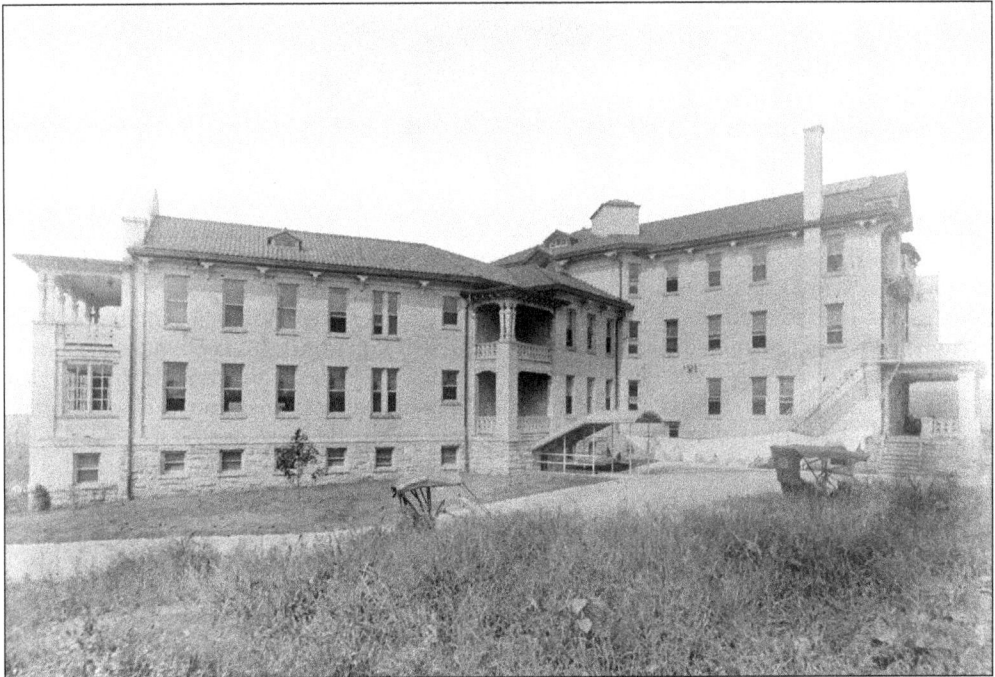

The most striking thing about this view of the rear of the completed hospital is the line of wash, hanging in the sun to dry. Now that sunshine has been replaced by the electric dryer, this centuries-old method of drying laundry seems quaint rather than what it really was—practical.

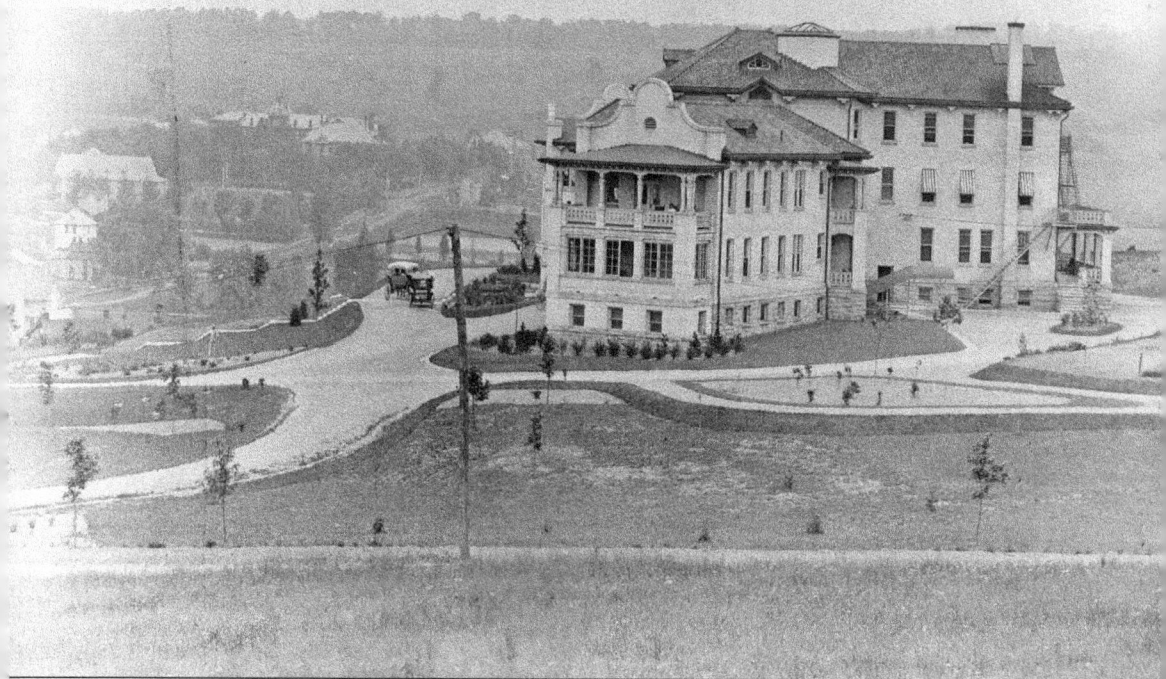

The images of the hospital site on these facing pages include many interesting details. This view of the east end and the rear of the building shows the fire escapes incorporated into the back porches, the covered entrance into the ground floor, and the top of the elevator shaft above the small porches near the ground floor entrance. On the drive, in front of the building, are a horse-drawn surrey and an early automobile, perhaps belonging to Dr. Fred Hutchison. In an interview conducted late in his career, Dr. Hutchison recalled that his auto appeared in an early photograph of the hospital. Juniata College and the Stone Church of the Brethren can be seen on the left side of the photograph, along with a few houses scattered along Warm Springs Avenue and other streets in this relatively undeveloped part of Huntingdon Borough.

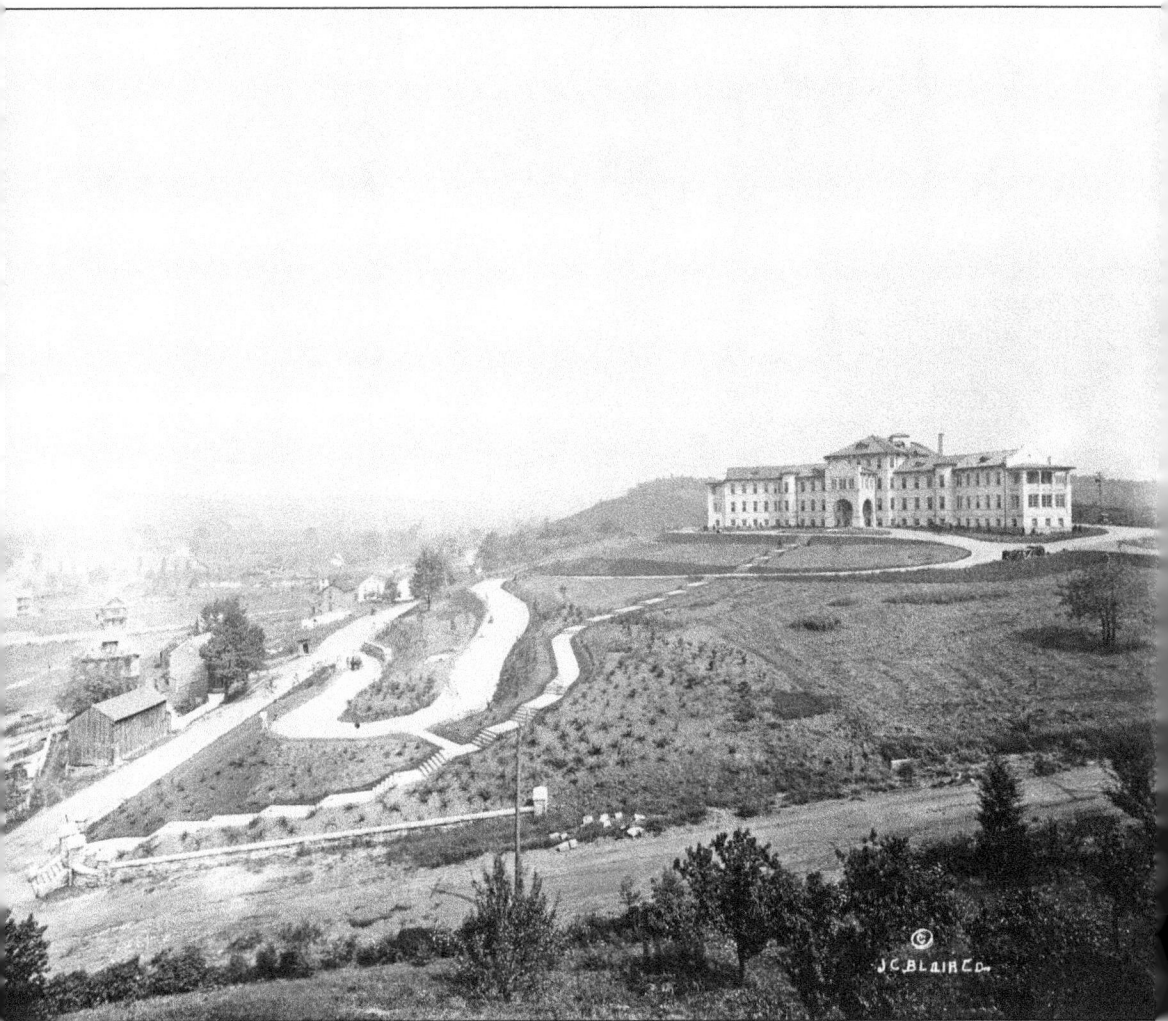

This more distant view, from a different angle, shows how the hospital dominated its elevated site before any trees had grown tall enough to obscure it. The long flight of steps leading up to it must have tested the stamina of all who approached on foot. The steep, rutted street in the foreground has not yet been paved with the yellow bricks that cover it today. In the middle distance, left, can be seen the pond that later became Benson Dairy's pond, from which they cut ice in winter. It is now the location of the Weis Market. Left of the pond is a row of trees, planted along the south side of the college athletic field.

23

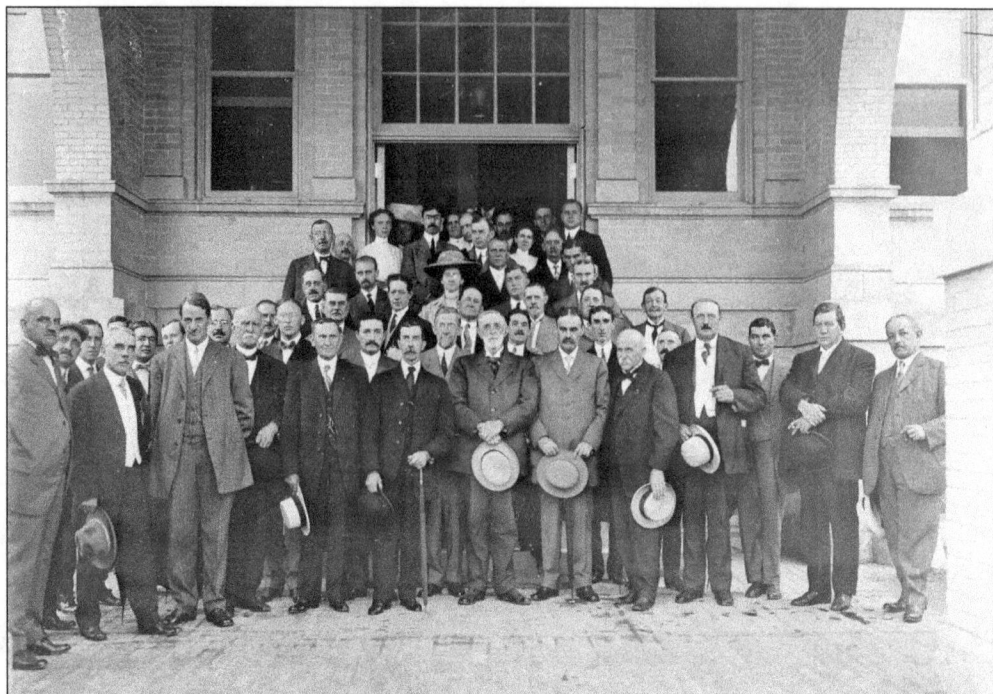

When construction of the hospital was complete and equipment in place, a Physicians' and Press Day was announced for August 24, 1911. Invited guests heard three speeches before touring the new building and gathering for a documentary photograph. Identified are: E. M. C. Africa, left; Dr. David P. Miller, center front; Dr. M. R. Evans, left of Dr. Miller; and I. Harvey Brumbaugh, second row, with center part and bushy brows.

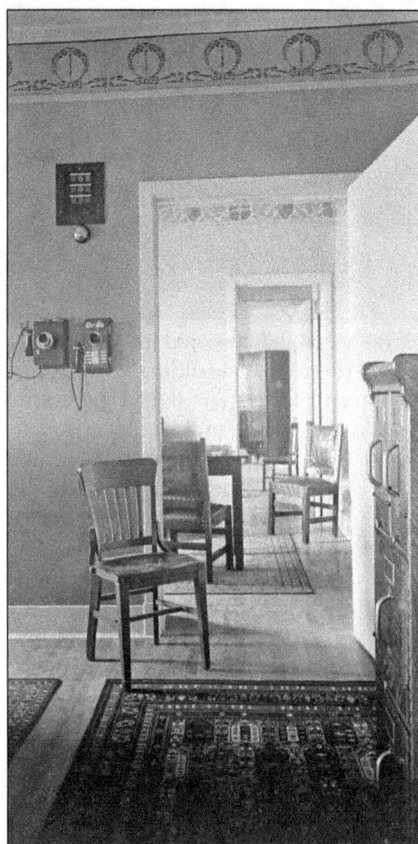

Before the invited guests toured the hospital, the J. C. Blair Company photographer captured images of what the physicians and press would see. Thus, we can join the group as the facilities, including this business office, are viewed for the first time. The views seen here were also offered as postcards to the public, who were invited to tour the building from August 28 to 30, 1911.

Identified as the library in the booklet printed to commemorate Physicians' and Press Day, this room may also have served as a conference or boardroom. It features a bold arts and crafts frieze and Mission-style furniture, both in fashion at the time.

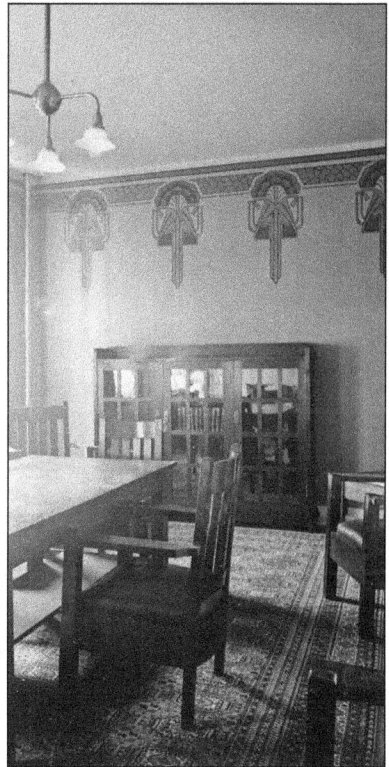

The hospital superintendent's position was always filled by a woman who was a registered nurse, and she occupied a spacious tower room furnished with a brass bed, double-mirrored dresser, writing desk, and wicker rocker. It is also likely that an armoire and washstand stood in the corner from which the image was taken.

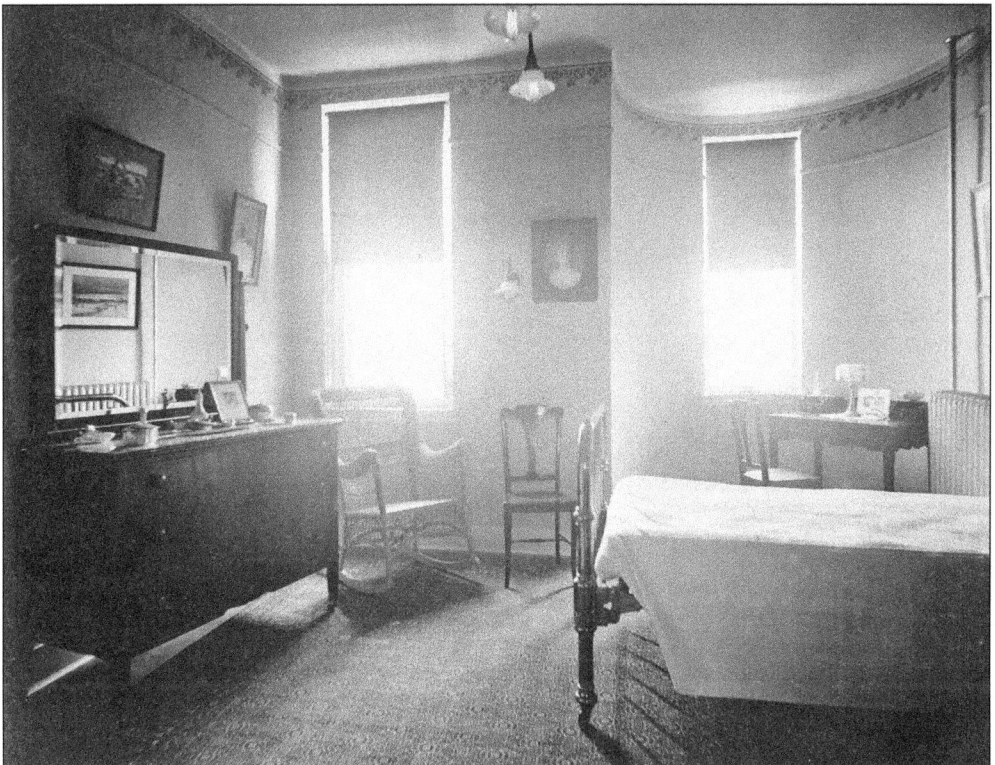

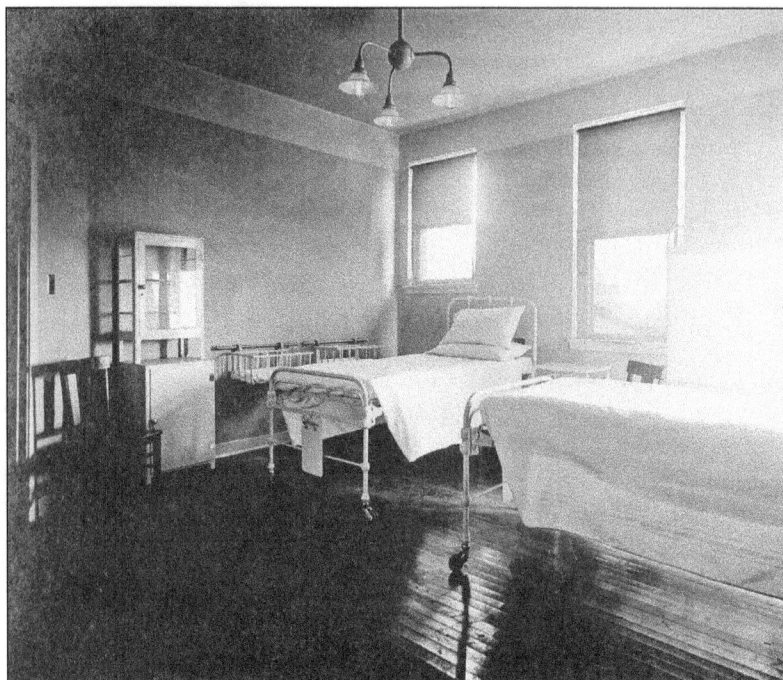

This two-bed maternity room is outfitted with white iron beds on casters, bassinets that hang from a wall-mounted rod, a movable privacy screen, and two straight chairs for the very restricted visitors allowed into maternity patients' rooms. The view out the window reveals that the room is located on the third floor, above the main entrance.

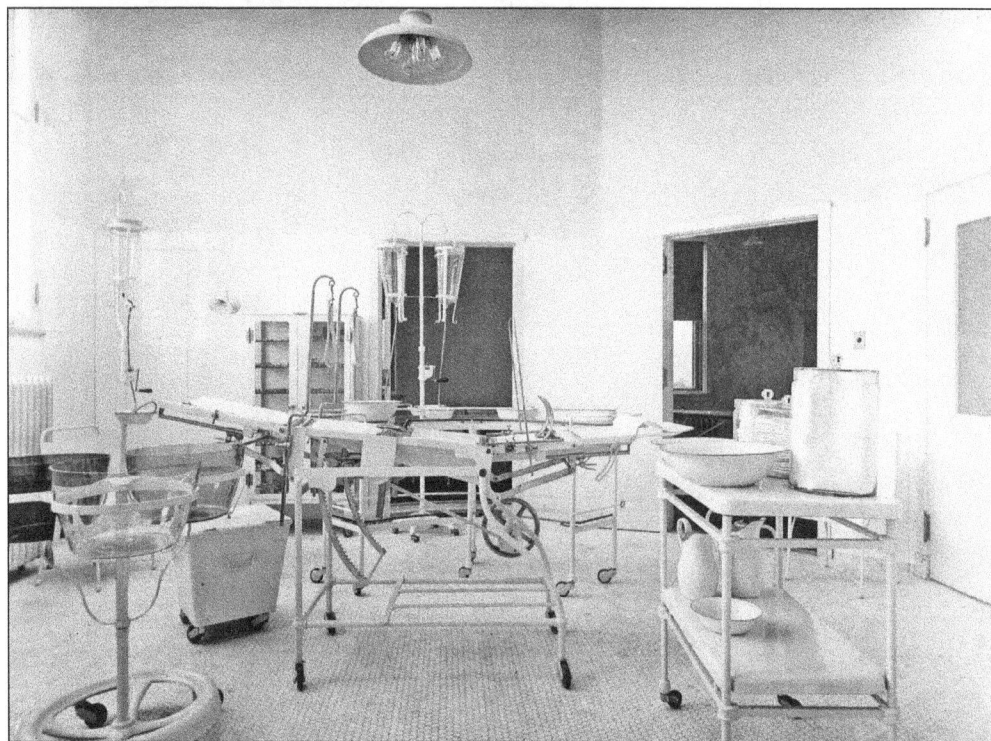

The delivery room fixtures are almost all on casters to allow whatever arrangement best suits the staff and the circumstances. Both ends of the delivery table are adjustable, and a narrow rod-like frame allows for draping the patient. The room is lighted by three large windows (seen in another view) and an overhead light that holds four early incandescent bulbs.

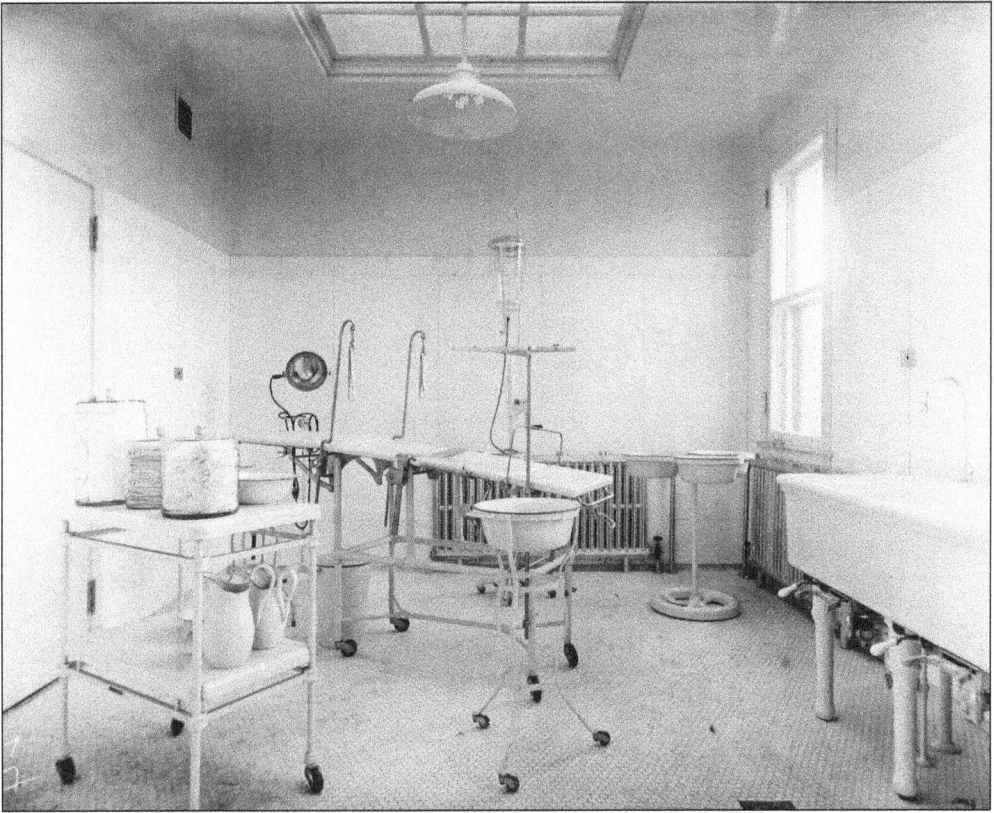

As in the delivery room, the operating room table, utility cart, and large basin are on casters, making it possible to arrange the room to suit the surgeon's requirements. The large porcelain sink has leg-operated levers that allow the staff to scrub without touching the faucets. Light is provided by a skylight, as well as an overhead fixture and a portable floodlight.

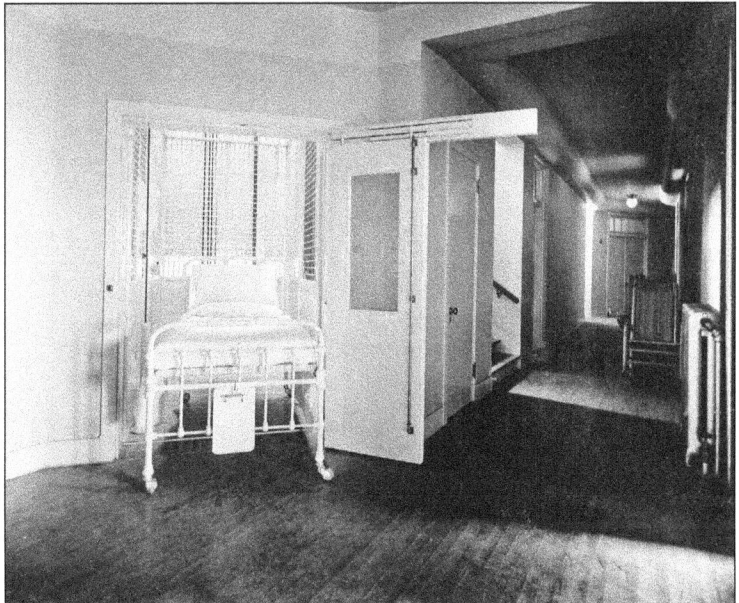

With the delivery and operating rooms on different floors from patients' rooms, an elevator was essential to the hospital's operation. The open-work walls of the elevator car would not meet present-day safety regulations but might have allayed fears of being stuck in an airless car.

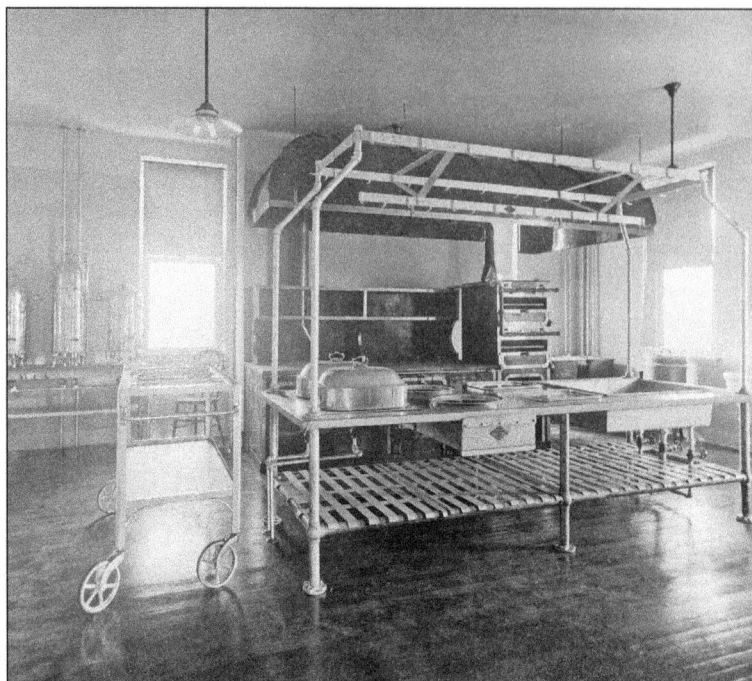

In certain respects, this utilitarian room has a lot of similarities to a modern institutional kitchen, except for the stove pipes emerging from the stove and the stacked ovens. Apparently they were coal-or wood-fired. The coffee urns, steam table, wheeled service cart, and rack for hanging pots have not changed radically in a century's time.

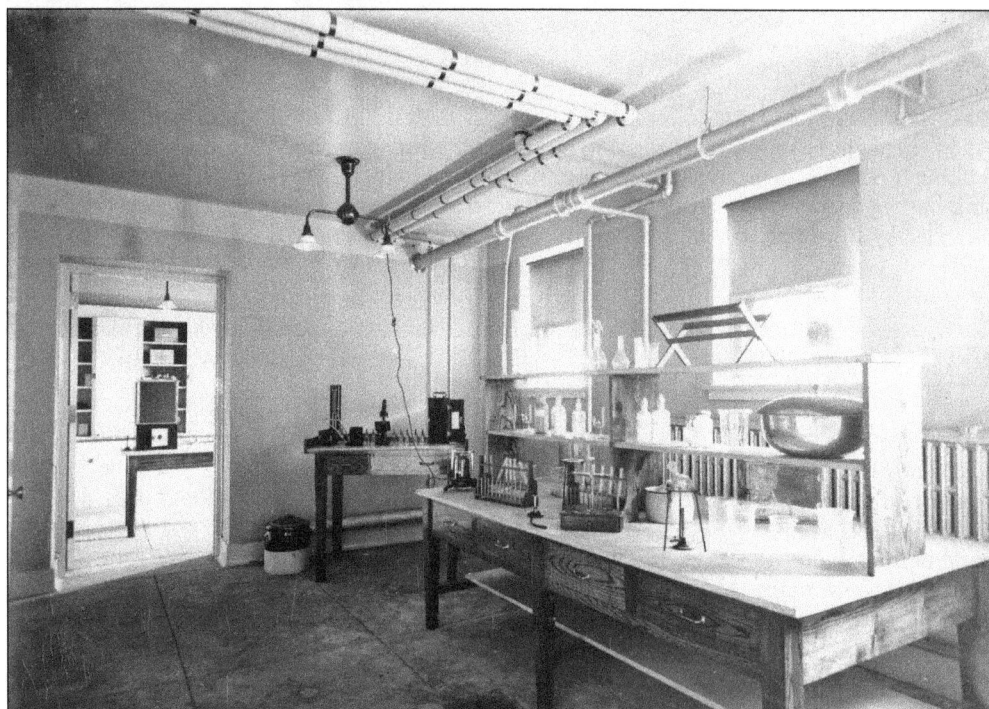

The germ theory of disease was not fully accepted until little more than a decade before the opening of J. C. Blair Memorial Hospital. This sparsely furnished laboratory indicates the new hospital intended to apply scientific analysis to their care of patients. The room is obviously located on the basement level of the building; notice the many pipes on the ceiling serving rooms on the floors above.

Three

AUXILIARY

Two years after J. C. Blair Memorial Hospital opened its doors, a Ladies' Auxiliary was organized. While mostly wives of doctors and trustees attended the first meeting, the group cast a wide net in the community, enlisting an amazingly large membership with annual dues of just $1.

It would be difficult to overstate the dedication and energy the Auxiliary brought to its mission of supporting the hospital financially, as well as looking out for patients' comfort and welfare and entertaining the young women enrolled in the nursing school. In the early years, the organization covered the hospital's annual deficit, began a long tradition of purchasing equipment for the hospital's use, and sewed and mended literally thousands of linens and patient garments.

Fund-raising in support of the organization to which they are attached is, of course, the major function of any auxiliary. The hospital Auxiliary members demonstrated their ability in this realm early on. Their Carnival of Nations in 1914 was the first in a long list of successful fund-raising events, enabling the hospital to purchase its first motorized ambulance.

Aware of the importance of wide community involvement in the hospital's support, the Auxiliary devised an innovative annual campaign at Easter to enlist schoolchildren and their families in collecting eggs for the hospital's use. The effort eventually spread from the immediate Huntingdon area to schools all over the county and hundreds of dozens of eggs were contributed.

Later projects included a band concert, publication of a popular book of members' recipes, and the long-running Charity Ball, begun in 1950 by the hospital but turned over to the Auxiliary within a few years. Volunteers in the snack bar and gift shop racked up countless hours. Radio and television connections in patient rooms were once fund-raising sources; cable television is now provided by the Auxiliary at no cost to patients. The organization's current activities reflect many of the same priorities that have guided the Auxiliary's projects throughout its history.

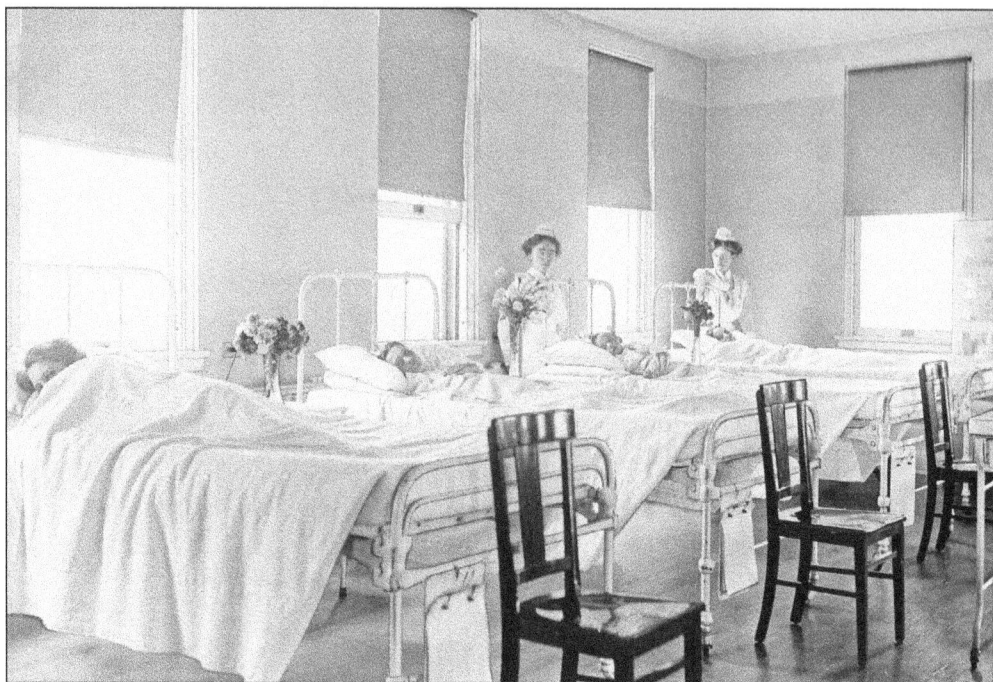

The flowers at every bedside were provided by the Auxiliary, which was dedicated in its early years to making each patient's hospital stay as pleasant and comfortable as possible. Members bought dozens of vases, which they filled with flowers from their own gardens. At Christmas and Easter, flowers were purchased to decorate the hospital, and money was contributed every summer to assure that ward patients could enjoy ice cream.

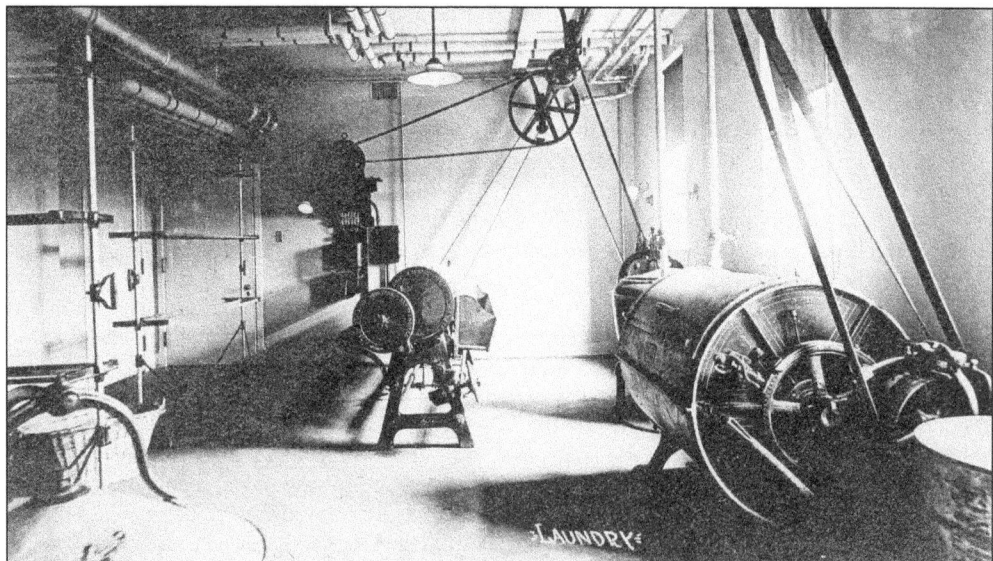

The hospital's original laundry equipment must have severely stressed the fabric of bedclothes and patient garments. Auxiliary members maintained a constant program of mending and sewing. In 1920, for example, the Red Cross donated material from which 54 bathrobes and kimonos were made, along with 33 blankets, 24 baby napkins, and 3 pneumonia jackets. In addition, the women mended 53 garments and assorted linens that year.

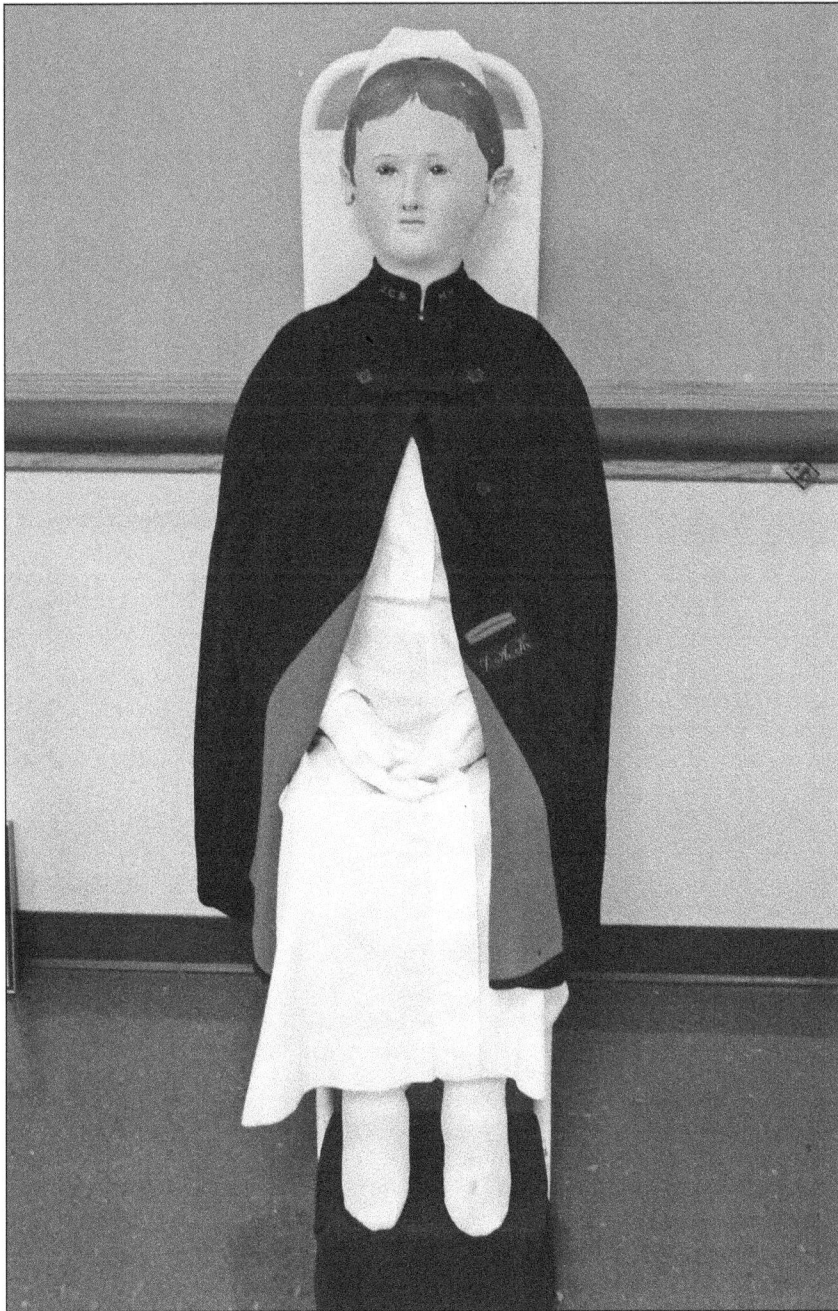

A committee of the Auxiliary was appointed June 9, 1914, to purchase a Chase doll on which student nurses could practice their developing skills. Chase dolls were manufactured by Martha Chase, who began by making dolls for her children and then went into business in her backyard to fill a Boston department store's order. Later the Chase Company produced baby dolls for educating new mothers and student nurses. Requested to make an adult model, Chase introduced dolls like this one in 1914. Nursing students named their dolls, dubbing many of them "Mrs. Chase." J. C. Blair students called their doll "Rosebud," for the rosebud mouth on her painted face. On display in the hospital, she now wears traditional nurse's garb. (Photograph by Linda Cutshall.)

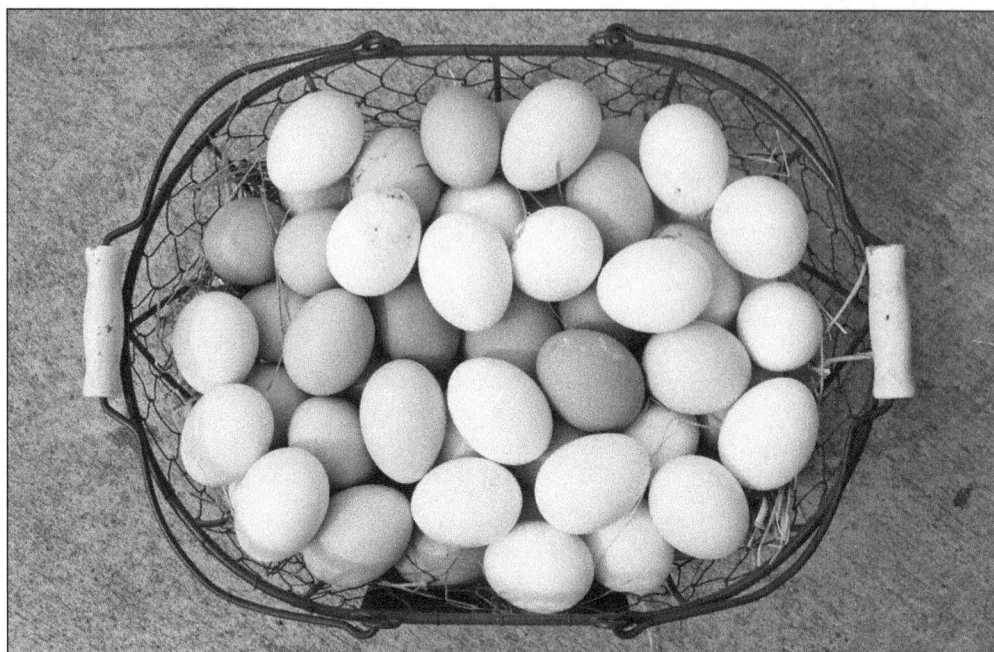

For 35 years, the Auxiliary asked school children to contribute eggs to the hospital at Easter. The first year's successful campaign, in 1914, yielded 120 dozen eggs. After expanding to include schools in areas where the branch auxiliaries were active—Mount Union, Lower Huntingdon County, and Alexandria-Petersburg—a high point was reached in 1944 when 790 dozen eggs were gathered in 16 different schools.

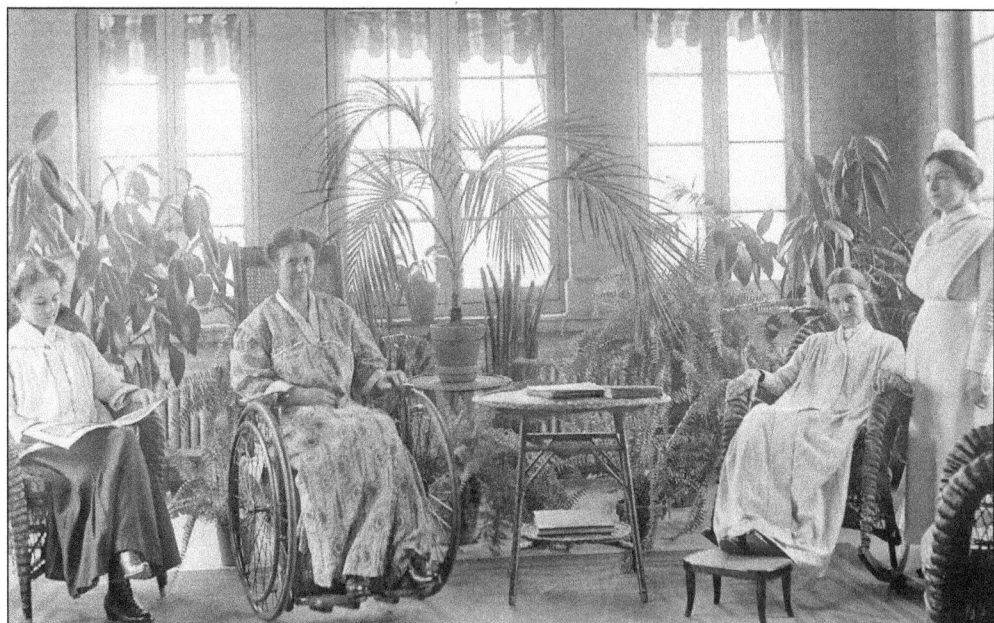

At a time when hospital stays might extend to a week or more, convalescing patients could enjoy the relaxing atmosphere of the solariums, which repeated Auxiliary efforts kept attractive and comfortable. The windows were of vita glass, which allowed the passage of ultraviolet rays, newly discovered to be effective in killing harmful microorganisms.

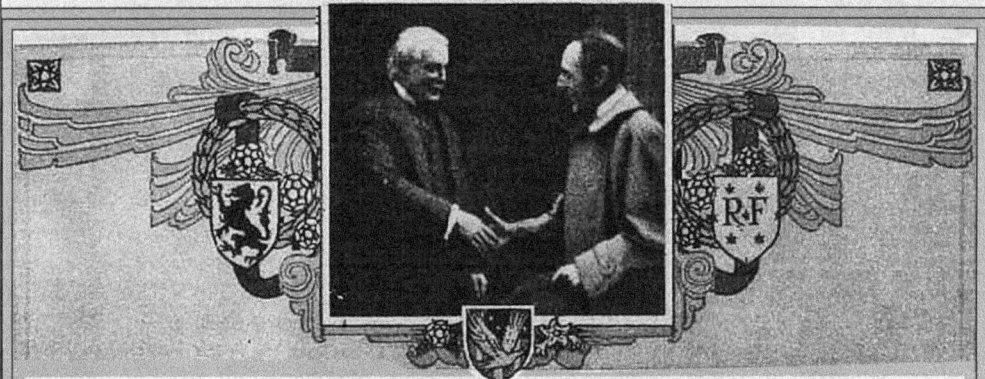

AT GRAND THEATRE

Huntingdon. 2 Days. Matinee Saturday
Friday and Saturday, July 11 and 12

DAVID LLOYD GEORGE, PRIME MINISTER OF ENGLAND
BIDDING GOD-SPEED TO DAVID WARK GRIFFITH
ON THE EVE OF HIS DEPARTURE FOR FRANCE

D. W. GRIFFITH'S
SUPREME TRIUMPH
HEARTS of the WORLD

The sweetest love story ever told
A romance of the great war
Battle scenes taken on the battle-fields of France
(Under auspices of the British and
French War Offices)

Prices, Nights, 8.00 P.M. 25c, 50c, $1.00, and $1.50
Prices, Matinee, 2.15 P.M. 25c, 50c, 75c, and $1.00

In 1919, Mrs. Thomas F. Bailey, an active Auxiliary member, entertained the student nurses at dinner and took them to the "moving pictures," where they may have seen D. W. Griffith's World War I film *Hearts of the World*. The Auxiliary was much involved in the students' leisure activities and, in response to a request from them in 1918, hired Ella Quinn to give them dancing lessons.

33

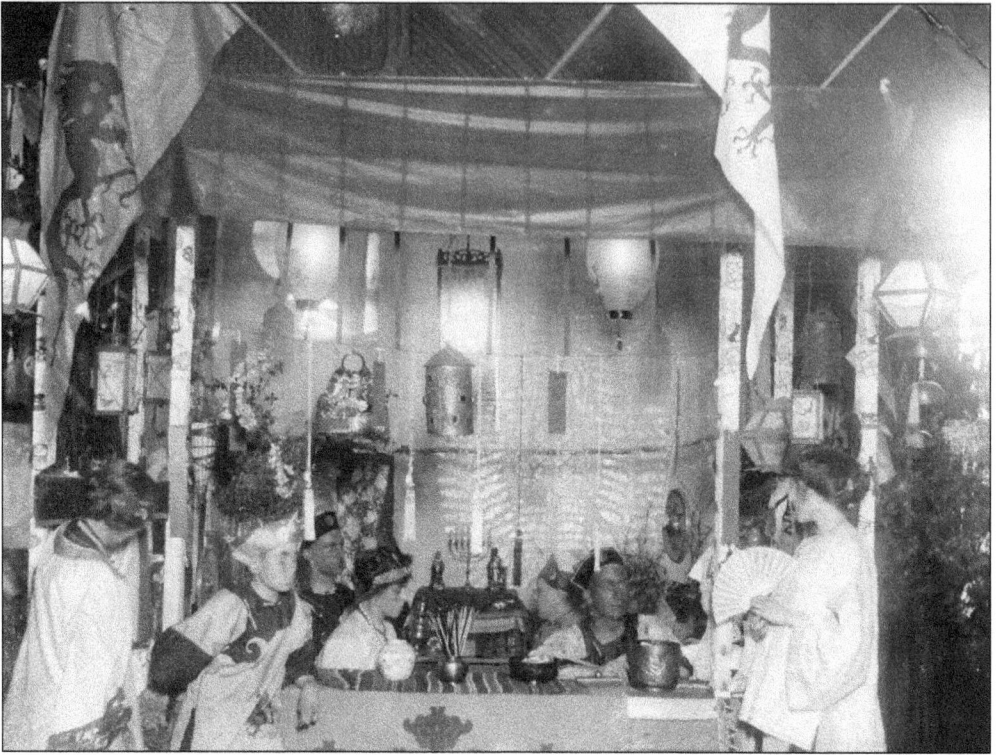

The Ladies' Auxiliary presented the Carnival of Nations in 1914 as a major fund-raiser toward the purchase of an ambulance. The three-day affair included booths representing 11 nations around the world, as well as two comic plays and a Frolic of Holidays. Mrs. Oscar H. Irwin (Elsie Black) headed the committee for China and is seen here (left of center, in profile) in their elaborate Chinese booth. Hundreds of prominent Huntingdon residents and young people performed in the plays, staffed the booths, and sang and danced in the Frolic held in the old Armory at the top of Seventh Street.

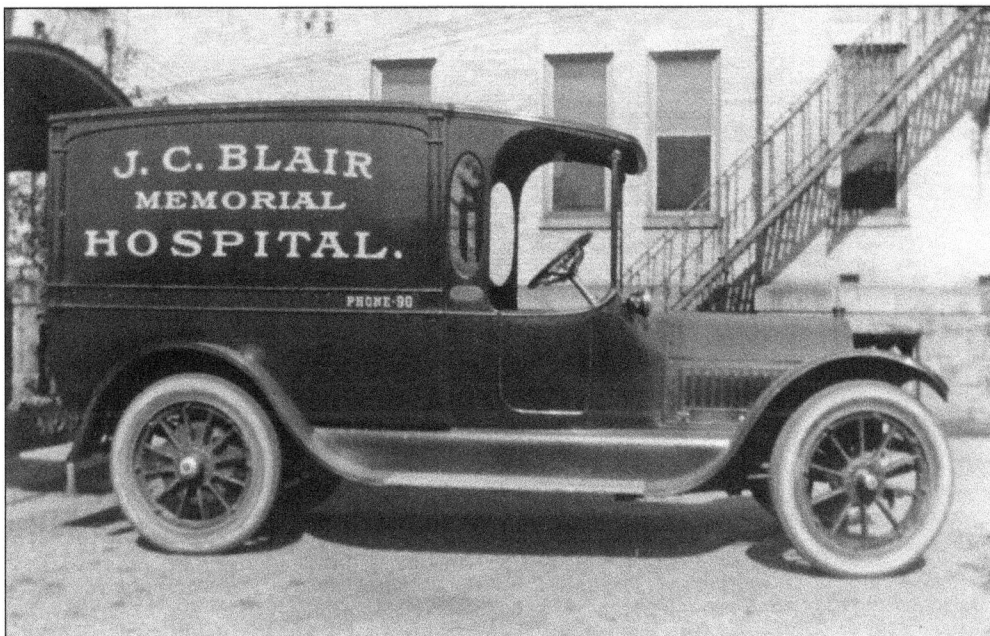

Of the $2,868.40 raised by the Carnival of Nations, the Auxiliary donated $2,000 to the ambulance fund to replace a horse-drawn ambulance donated by the Pennsylvania Railroad in 1911. The vehicle's oval side windows and columns framing the name panel indicate that this model, perhaps a Cadillac, could also be ordered for use as a hearse. (Courtesy of Alice Hurwitz.)

Four members of the hospital's board of trustees appeared in the cast of *Trial for Breach of Promise*, one of the entertainments presented during the Carnival of Nations. Principals in the play were Blanche Black, as the innocent young thing, and Huntingdon dentist Dr. W. C. Wilson as the "heartless wretch" who done her wrong.

Saturday, May 9th, 1914

TRIAL FOR BREACH OF PROMISE

ARAMINTA CLOVERTOP
vs.
J. BARRYMORE de BROWN-SMYTHE } May Term, 1914.

JURORS

A. Hardcase	Mr. C. H. Miller
M. T. Head	Mr. H. E. Butz
Hans Zweilager	Mr. Robt. Steel
U. R. Greenhorn	Mr. S. A. Hamilton
Chow Chow Sing Sing	Mr. Thos. J. Gipple
I. M. Deadbeat	Mr. H. W. Koch
Hannibal Washington Napoleon Snowball	Rev. E. N. Thomas
Ichabod Numbskull	Mr. O. H. Irwin
N. Swindler	Mr. John Grove
Pat Moriarity	Mr. W. S. Conrad
Sandy McNab	Mr. Frank Stewart
P. D. Quick	Mr. Chester Fetterhoof

LITIGANTS

PLANTIFF
Miss Araminta Clovertop (A country blossom)   Miss Blanche Black
DEFENDANT
Mr. J. Barrymore de Browne-Smythe   -   -   Dr. W. C. Wilson
(A handsome heartless wretch)

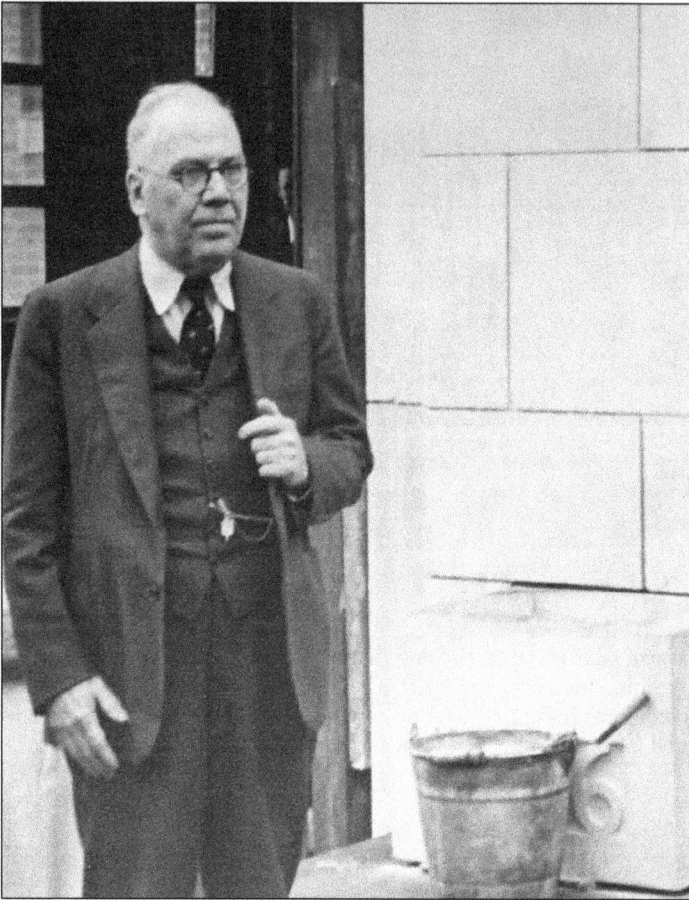

Dr. Willis Gatch, inventor of the three-part adjustable hospital bed, was photographed at the laying of the cornerstone for the Gatch Clinical Building, at the Indiana University School of Medicine in 1936. That same year, Auxiliary members were told by Helen Stabler, supervisor of nurses, of the great need to supply the hospital with Gatch beds. The Auxiliary responded by ordering six of the beds through C. H. Miller Hardware at a cost of $228. In the next five years, the Auxiliary continued purchasing beds until all of the hospital's old-fashioned beds had been replaced. (Both, courtesy of IUPUI University Library Ruth Lilly Special Collections and Archives.)

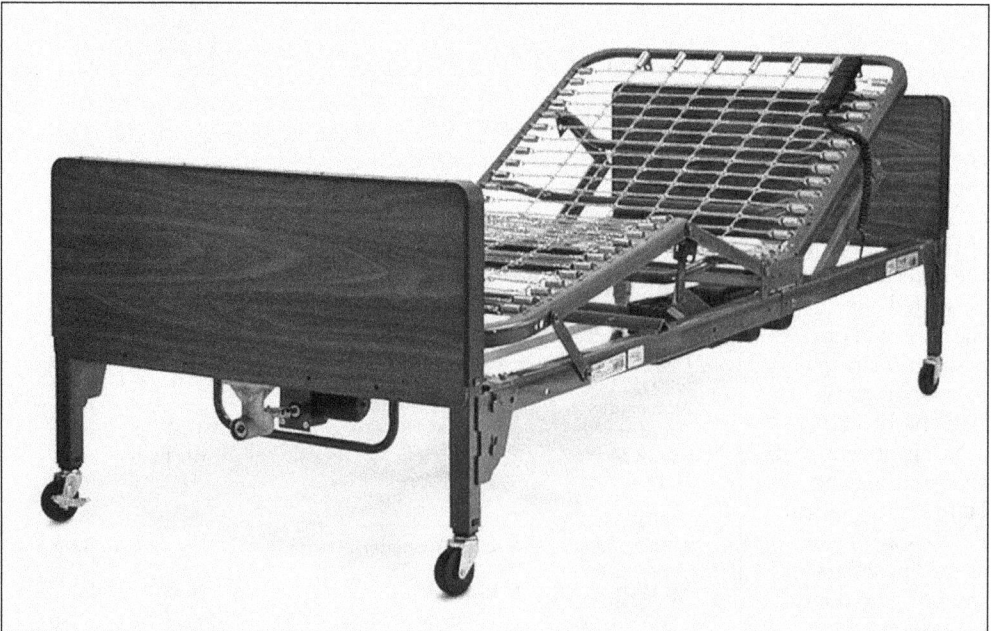

PERSONAL APPEARANCE
THE UNITED STATES
NAVY BAND
LCdr CHARLES BRENDLER, USN, Conductor

The World's Finest

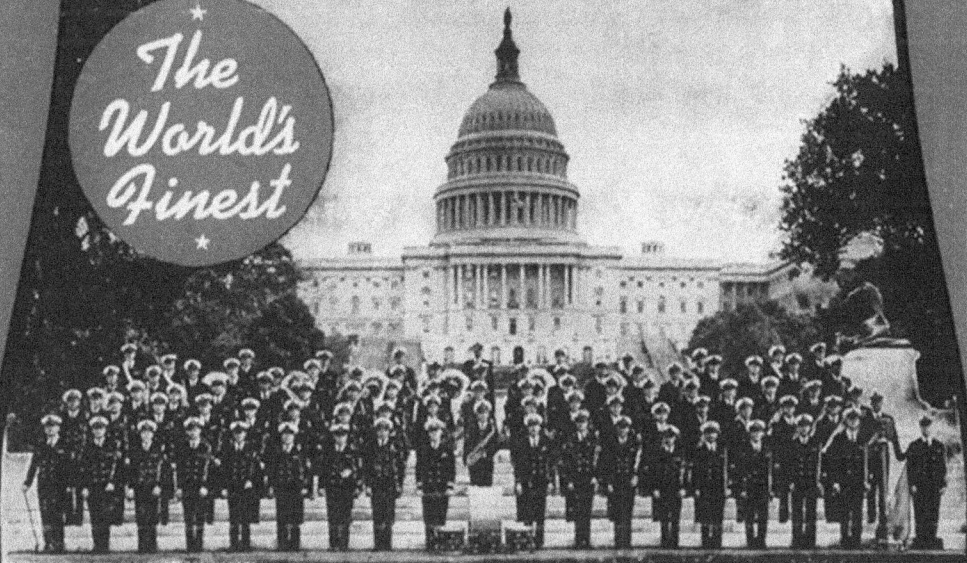

The U. S. Navy Band on Steps of Nation's Capitol

Saturday, May 21, 1948
Performances at 2:00 p.m. & 8:15 p.m.
War Veterans Field, Huntingdon
Sponsored by
the Auxiliary to J.C. Blair Memorial Hospital

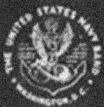

ANNUAL TOUR APPROVED BY THE PRESIDENT
Gib SANDEFER, Concert Tour Director — Suite 1092 National Press Building, Washington 4, D. C.

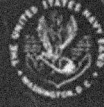

This Auxiliary fund-raiser packed the bleachers for both the afternoon and evening performances. Seventeen outstanding musicians from Huntingdon County schools played with the band at the matinee, for which the Huntingdon and Broad Top Mountain Railroad ran an excursion train from Hopewell to Huntingdon. The audience was estimated at 3,000; ticket prices were $1.50 for adults, 30¢ for elementary pupils, and 60¢ for high school students. Funds raised covered the $1,700 cost of the band and still yielded a profit of $1,215.16.

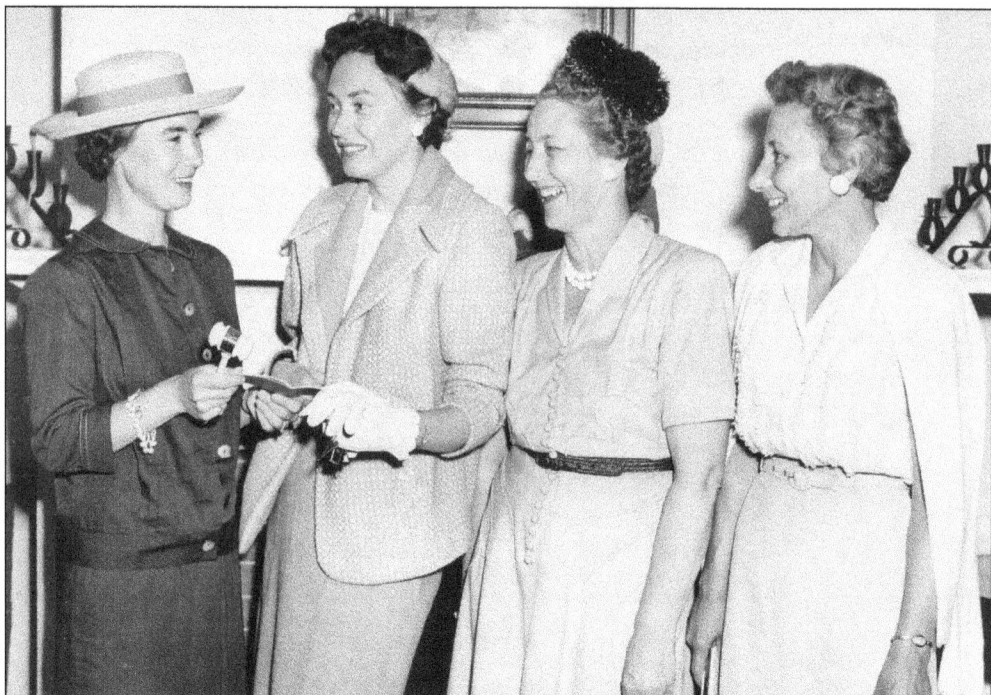

In June 1957, Mrs. D. A. Reese (left), newly installed president of the Auxiliary, received congratulations from Mrs. Frederic H. Steele (second from left), Mrs. James Ulsh (third from left), and Mrs. F. Glenn Westbrook. More than 50 years ago, women still wore hats and gloves to afternoon events, although they were becoming optional, and newspapers understood that young matrons were properly identified by their husbands' names, not their own.

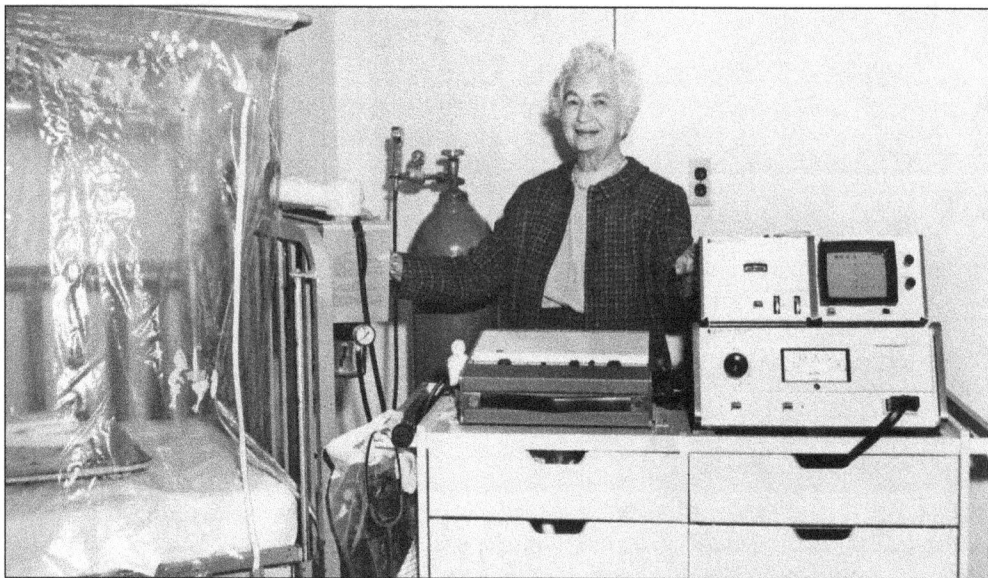

Branches of the Auxiliary in areas of the county outside of Huntingdon have played an important role in fulfilling the organization's traditional functions. Mrs. John A. Kunz, a moving force in the Alexandria-Petersburg (later Juniata Valley) branch, is pictured with an oxygen tent contributed by that group.

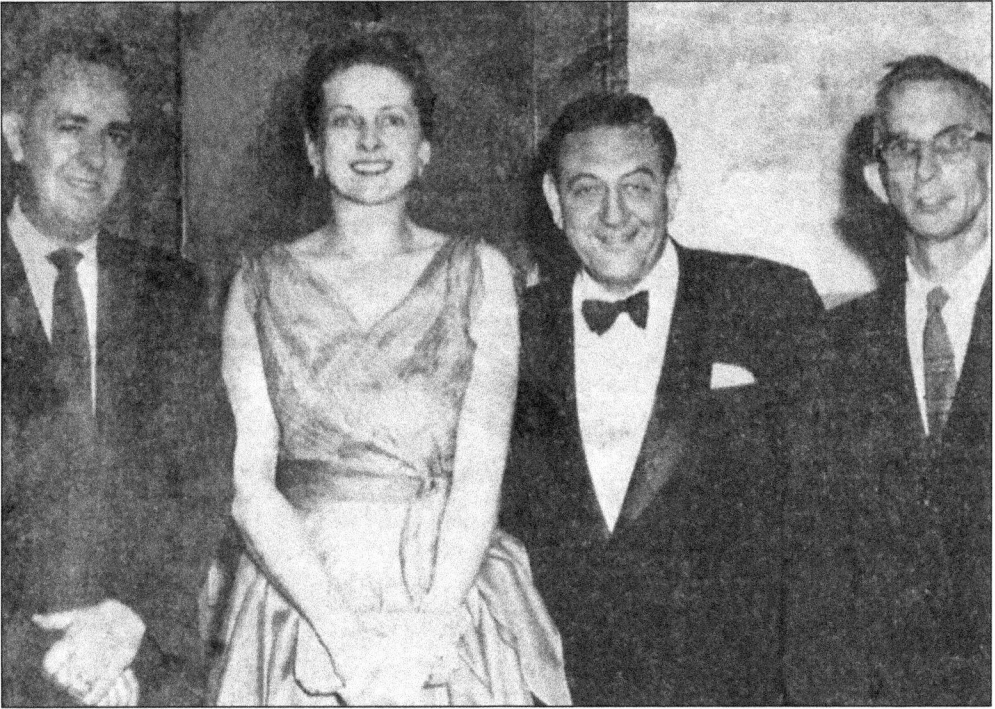

A record-breaking crowd danced to the music of Guy Lombardo and His Royal Canadians in Juniata's Memorial Gymnasium at the 1958 Charity Ball, the first to feature a band of the first rank. Chairs for the event were Attorney and Mrs. Warren Yocum (left) and Mr. and Mrs. William Germann (Mr. Germann, right), seen here with the famed bandleader, who played the "sweetest music this side of heaven."

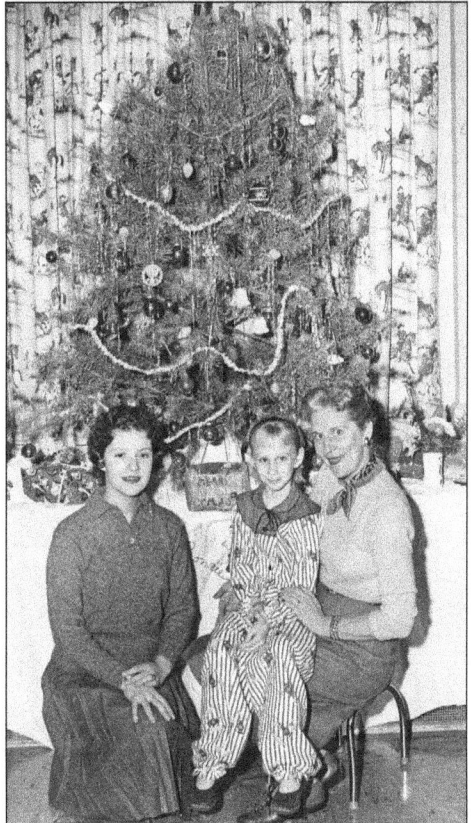

Following a long Auxiliary tradition, decorations were provided in 1959 by members of the TeenAge Auxiliary, who trimmed Christmas trees throughout the hospital. Mrs. H. Evan Huston (right), advisor to the teenagers, posed with Gay Clark, president of the teen group, and patient Sandra Kay Blair.

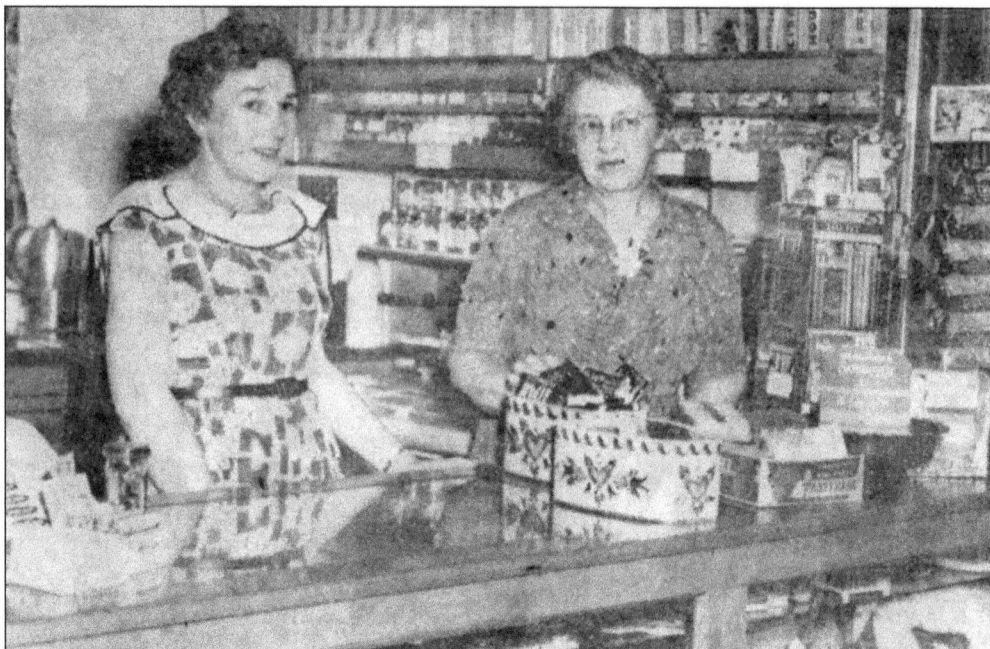

After construction of the 1950 building, the Auxiliary opened a snack bar and gift shop in the corridor connecting the two buildings. Mrs. Alva Walton (left) and Mrs. H. H. Nye, who chaired the project, are seen here behind a showcase displaying gift items. Volunteers staffed the snack bar, and all proceeds benefited the hospital.

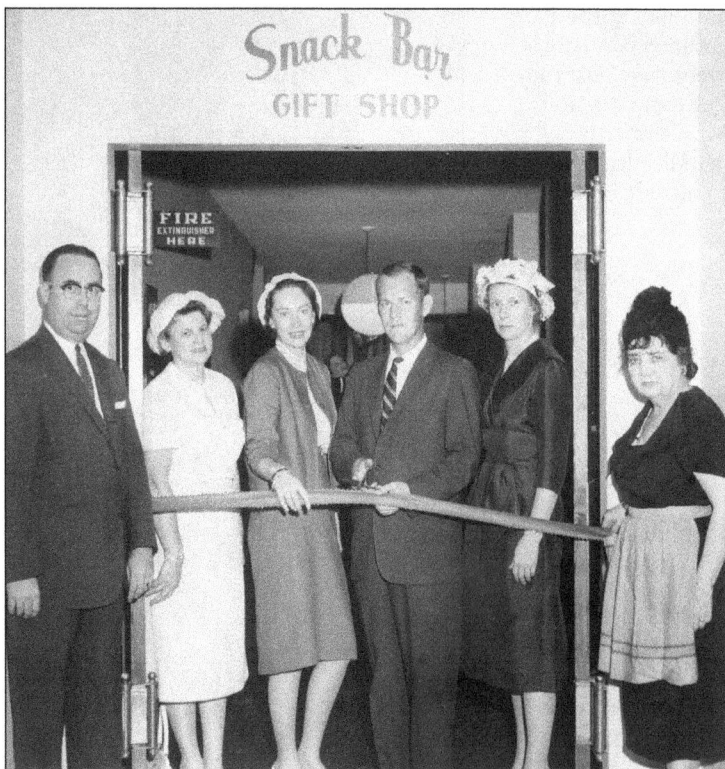

The Auxiliary's snack bar was relocated in 1960 to the ground floor of the 1950 building, where the cafeteria is now. Participants in the ribbon cutting were, from left to right, administrator Richard Cummings; Mrs. J. Robert Vastine, Shamokin; Mrs. Frederic H. Steele, Auxiliary president; William C. Huston, board president; Mrs. William U. Todd Jr., first vice president; and Mrs. John D. Pennington, hospitality chair.

The pillow radio was one of many projects the Auxiliary promoted to make a patient's hospital experience more pleasant. Tokens from the machine seen here purchased minutes of playing time from the radio affixed to the headboard of the bed. The patient listened through the round speaker placed under the pillow. (Photograph by Linda Cutshall.)

As television became ubiquitous in the 1950s and 1960s, patients expected a set in every room. Administrator Richard Cummings (left), auxiliary president Mrs. Frederic H. Steele, and an unidentified man are seen here with a new wall-hung set. The Auxiliary still provides free cable hookups in all patient rooms at a cost of nearly $8,000 annually.

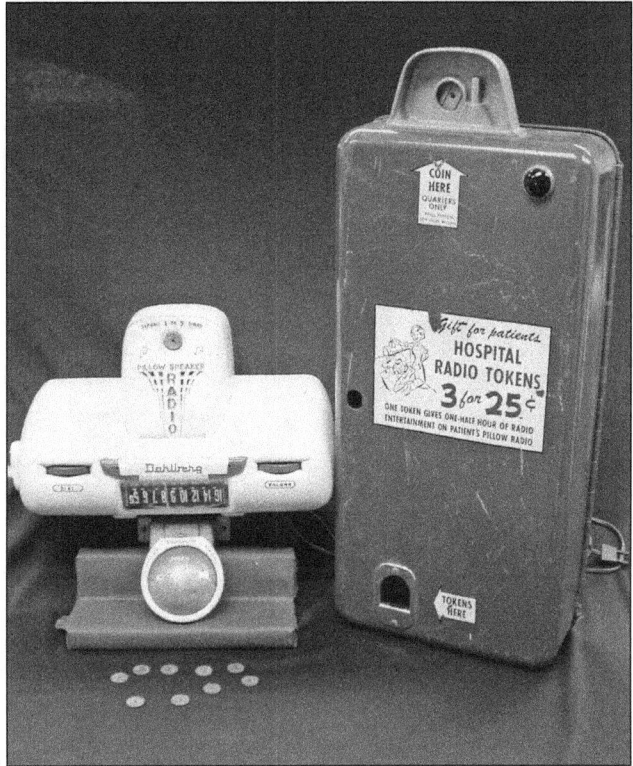

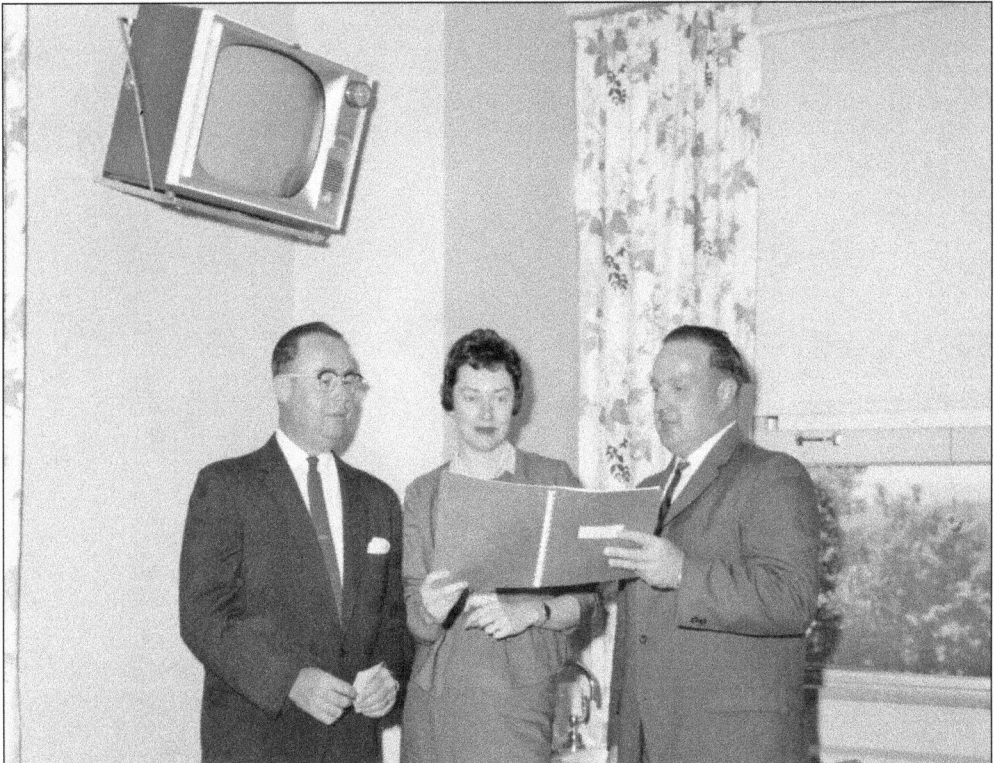

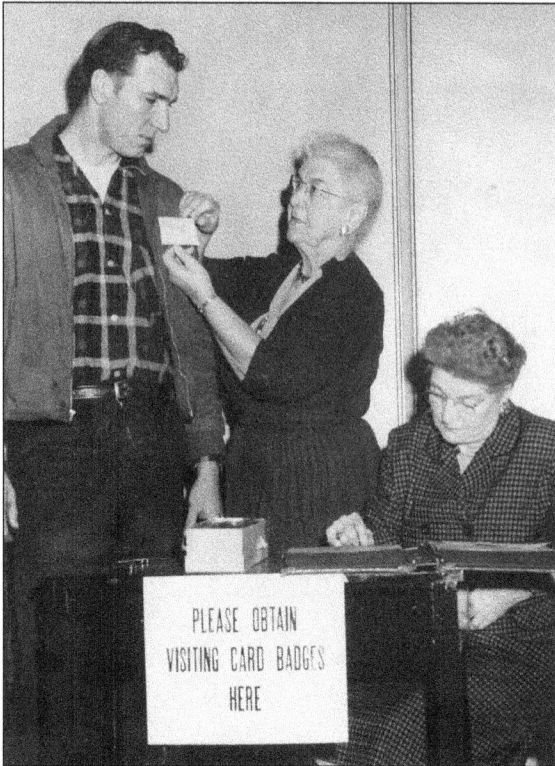

For many years, the Auxiliary has served on the front line of the interface between the hospital and the public, greeting and directing visitors and outpatients to destinations within the somewhat confusing maze of hallways, floors, and elevators. In 1960, Ellen McCulley, retired superintendent of nurses, pinned the first visitor badge on William Carolus of Petersburg as Ruth Smathers looked on. At the familiar area below where the pink-smocked Auxiliary volunteers now preside, Claire Todd, a longtime stalwart of the organization, places a telephone call for a visitor.

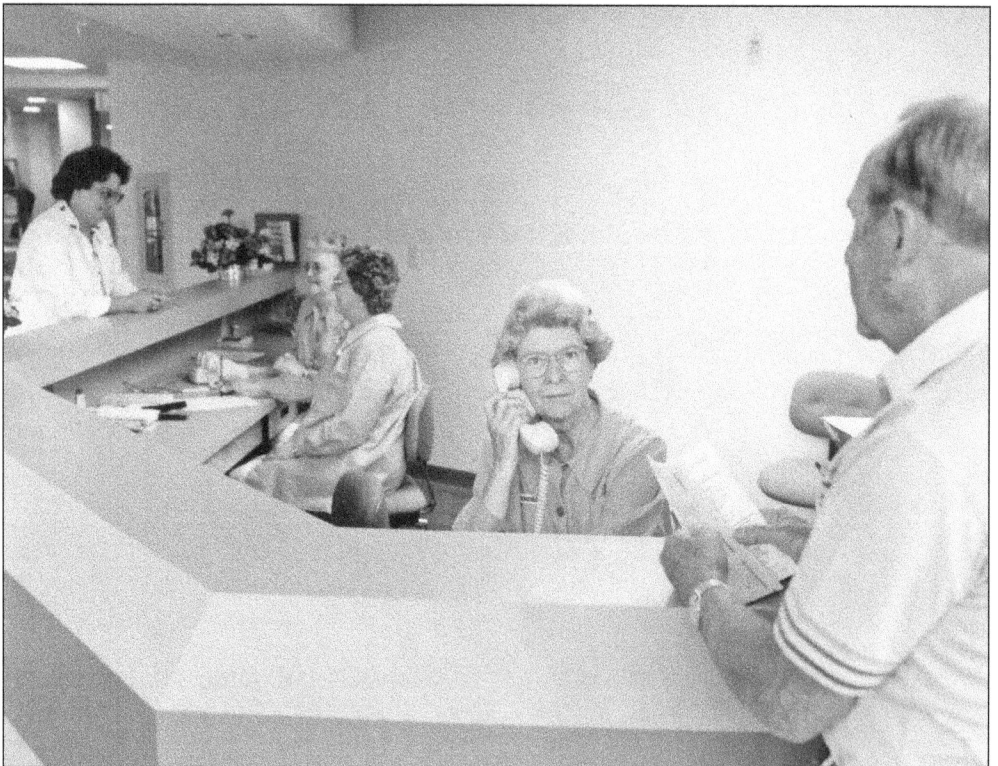

In 1960, the Lower Huntingdon County Auxiliary purchased hydrotherapy equipment, which their president, Mrs. E. L. Mills, presented to administrator Richard Cummings. Patients were immersed to the waist in 60 gallons of constantly moving water, which stimulated muscles and circulation. Used earlier to rehabilitate polio patients, physical therapists were finding other conditions that benefited from such treatment.

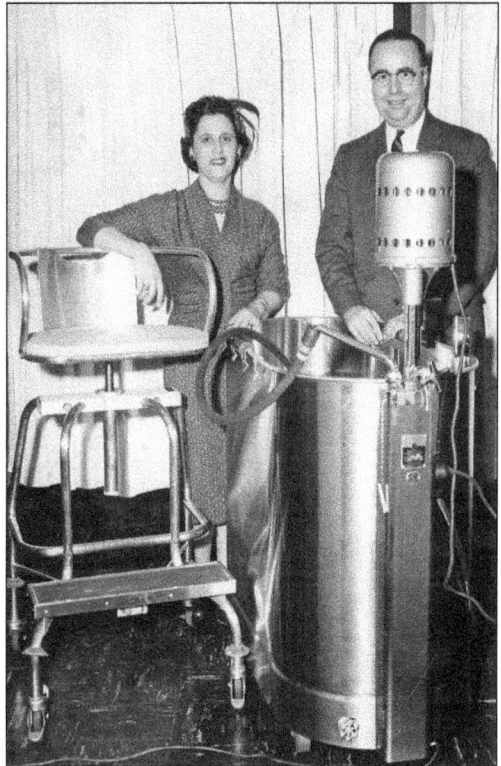

The Juniata Valley branch of the Auxiliary, represented by Mrs. John Kunz (third from left) and Mary Rush, presented a Robinson Orthopedic Stretcher to the Juniata Valley Ambulance Association in 1967. William Myers (left) and Glenn Metz accepted the gift.

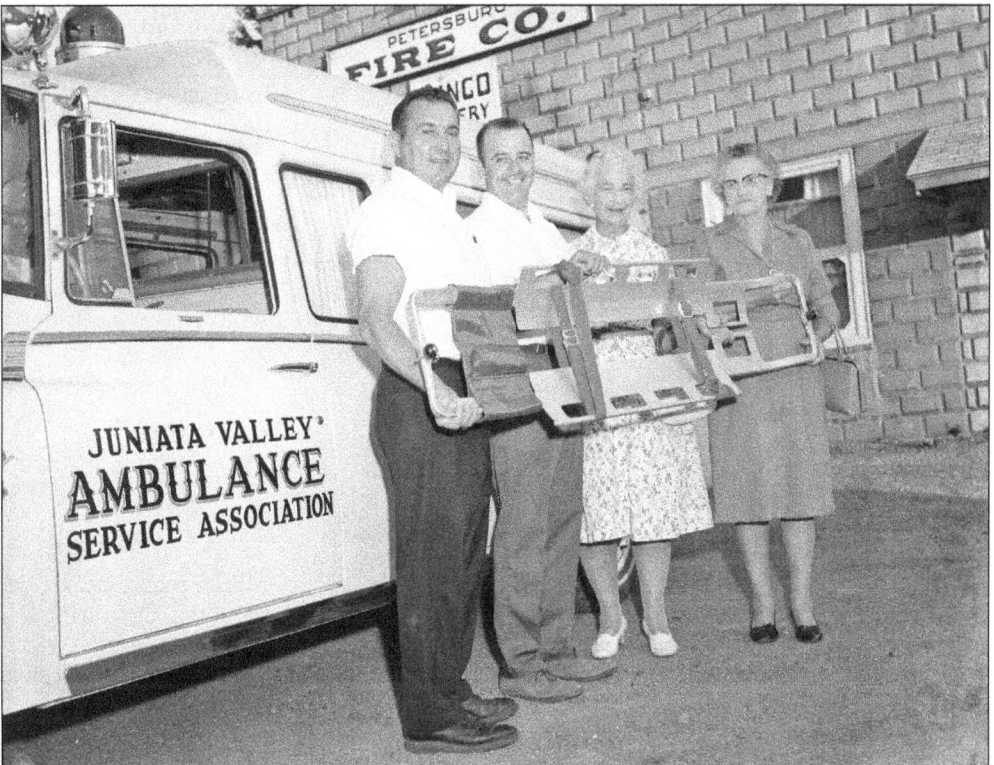

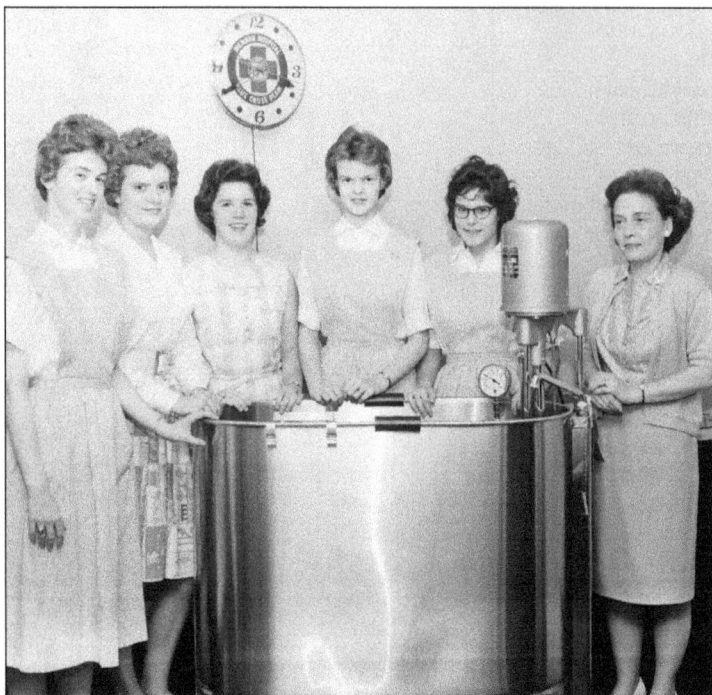

The Future Nurses of America club at Huntingdon Area High School (HAHS), organized by school nurse Elizabeth Shenefelt in 1961, served as candy stripers at the hospital, logging 2,004 hours of service that year. Photographed in 1962 with Auxiliary president Christine Schucker (right) were, from left to right, Sue Reynolds, Betty Jones, Carol Hirst, Barbara Porter, and Mary Terrizzi. Eight members of the HAHS Class of 1962 were accepted into nursing school.

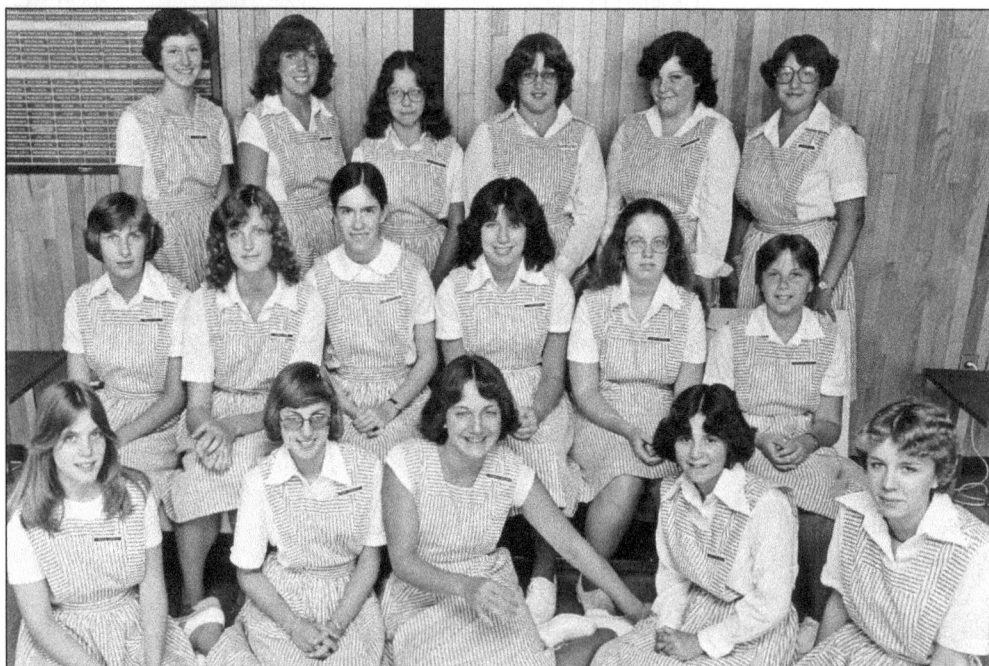

By the mid-1970s, the candy stripers were no longer all future nurses but any young women who volunteered their time and skills. Recognized in a newspaper photograph were, from left to right, (first row) Elaine Norris, Cynde Margritz, Barbara Slawson, Vicki Grinnell, and Sallye Margritz; (second row) Becky Kyper, Karen Elder, Mary Kay Miller, Rita Moran, Jane Weyant, and Polly Price; (third row) Kim Rinker, Elisabeth Kunz, Ann Hoffmaster, Cheryl Thornton, Sylvia Shope, and Pam Cella.

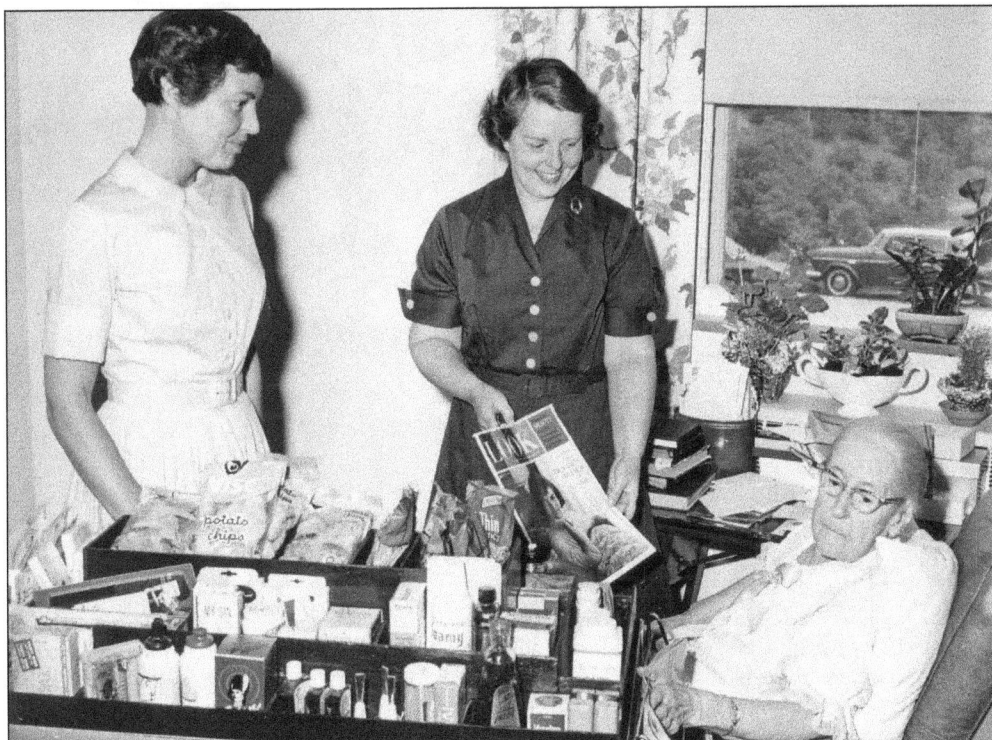

A cart selling necessities and gifts, seen here in the 1970s, began circulating through the hospital in 1948. Auxiliary members took the cart on its rounds and contributed toiletries, washcloths, crayons, and coloring books to stock "Liza," as it was affectionately called.

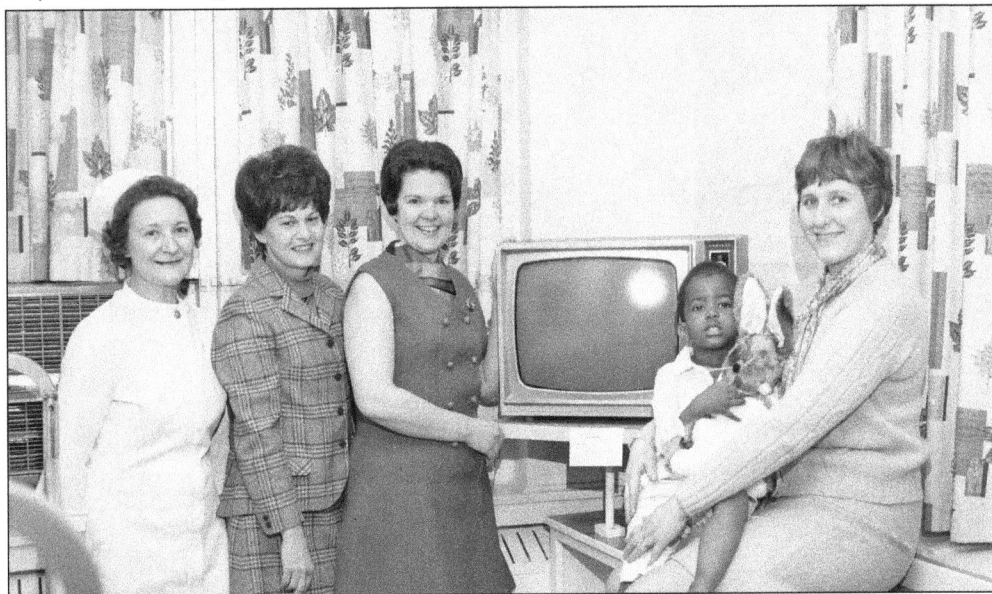

An Auxiliary project in 1970 brought a color television set to the pediatrics department. This photograph of the presentation finds committee chair Mrs. Richard Brown (right) holding patient Derrick Smith as longtime pediatric nurse Frances Hawn (left), Mrs. Forrest MacDonald (second from left), and Mrs. David Kunz look on.

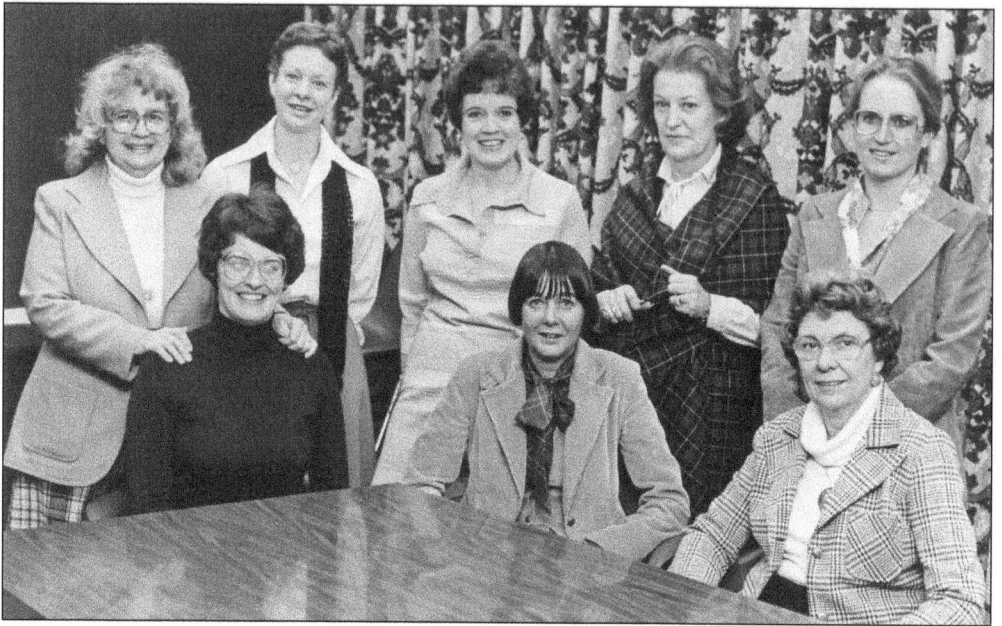

The Auxiliary has always been blessed with active members to carry its projects forward. Fitting that mold are members from the 1970s seen here. From left to right are (first row) Carol Cook, Mary Ellen Rosenhoover, and Claire Todd; (second row) Faye Mosser, Pam Thompson, Peggy Meloy, Nancy Rao, and Lynne Bayer. Rao and Thompson served the organization as president in the 1970s; Bayer and Cook in the 1980s.

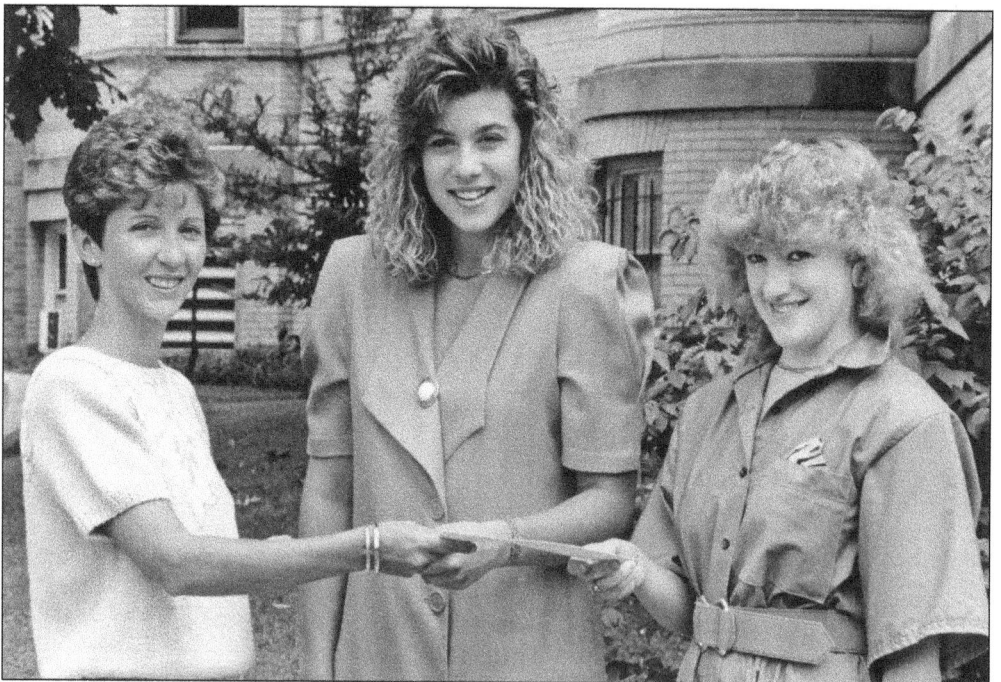

Since 1975, the Auxiliary has made scholarship awards to children of hospital employees to enable them to pursue further education. In 1989, Ellen Garner (left) presented checks to Melissa Bizak (center) and Ellen Nebgen, daughters of J. C. Blair nurses Leigh Bizak and Pat Nebgen.

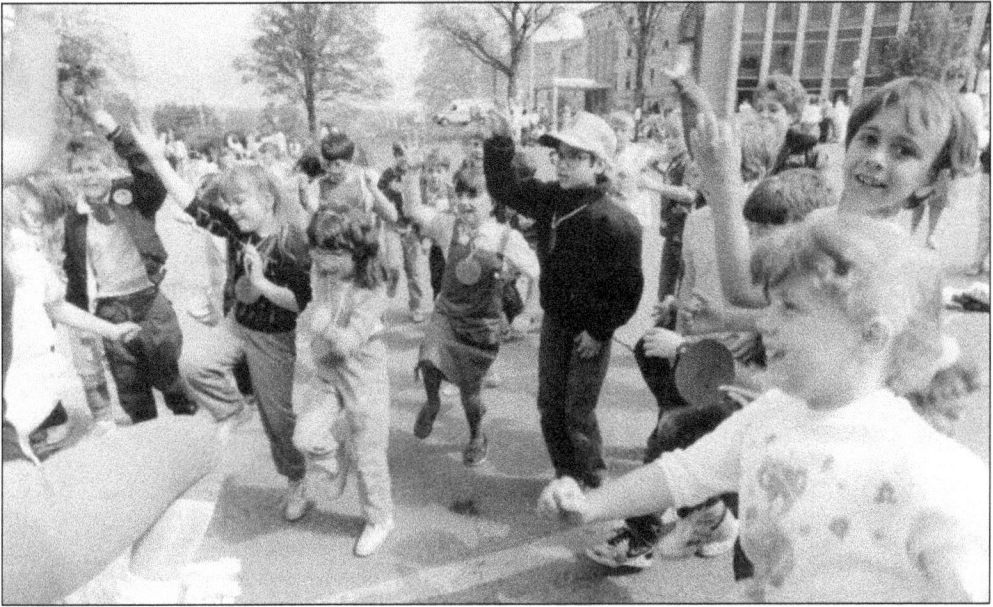

At the annual Children's Health Fair sponsored by the Auxiliary and the hospital, second and third graders are invited to spend a day at the hospital. They enjoy a program of educational activities designed to teach them important health principles, all while having fun. To judge by this photograph, the day was a great success.

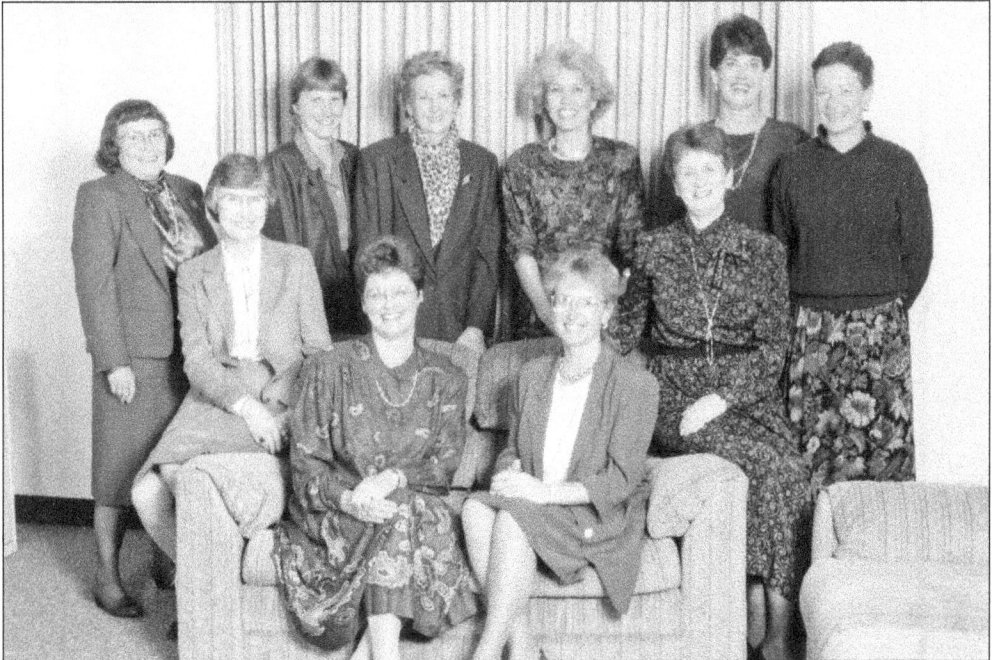

Thirty-five years of Auxiliary history are represented in this group portrait of 10 past presidents. From left to right are (first row) June Reese (1957–1959), Carol Cook (1987–1989), Lynne Bayer (1983–1985), and Donna King (1969–1971); (second row) Christine Schucker (1961–1963), Barbara Thomas (1981–1983), Lenore Conley (1977–1979), Rebecca Newton (1985–1987), Pat Bowman (1989–1991), and Pam Thompson (1979–1981).

IN TRIBUTE TO THE GRADUATES OF THE
J. C. BLAIR MEMORIAL HOSPITAL SCHOOL OF NURSING

Class of 1914
Anna Rachel Garner
Lucy Hamilton Coughton
Blanche Isenberg Parks
Elsie Lightner
Lida McAfee Leonard

Class of 1915
Alice Holden Green
Mary Isenberg Volpe
Mildred Stratford Shaffer

Class of 1916
Grace Chisolm Mueller
Edith Earl Care
Miriam Foust Hallin
Reba Leader Lucas
Mildred Neff

Class of 1917
Janet Bayley
Ethel Hooten
Jane McIntyre Hamilton
Fae Painter Brown
Gladys Stratford Lampman

Class of 1918
Helen Stewart Grey
Mary Krepps Shelley
Gladys Zerbe Miller
Beatrice Wright
Charlotte Vaughn Lowther
Etta Smith Steel

Class of 1919
Pearl Wilt Harris
Greta Weston Trohalakis
Mary Chilcote Huey
Almyra Keith Miller

Class of 1920
Bessie Shoemaker Van Triese
Wilda Doubles Woodring
Edna Boober Boyd
Julia Craig
Jane Dougherty
Louise Hartman Plasan

Class of 1921
Martha Mann Maguire
Martha Zimmerman

Class of 1922
Ruth Snyder Havens
Miriam Irvin Miller
Mary Smith Endres
Emma Zimmerman Landel
Blanche McDivitt Hoover
Myrtle Mosser Vandivert
Mattie Brown Tate
Mary Stever Miller
Valra McIntyre Boyer

Class of 1923
Elda Rhine Kitting
Violet Grove Hall
Lillian Grove

Class of 1924
Ethel Harshbarger Henderson
Jennie Rorabaugh

Class of 1925
Esther Bigelow Bradley
Pearl Hamilton
Mildred Isenberg Rhine
Inez Peek McIlroy
Pauline Reed Edwards
Ethel Gardner Morton
Mary Remmy Hohman
Minerva Shellenberger Lawrence
Thelma Showalter Miller
Pearl Mowery Snyder

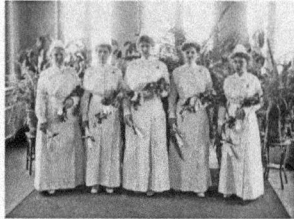

Class of 1914

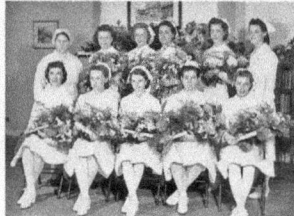

Class of 1940

Class of 1926
Virgie Moist Doyen
Harriet Lehman Miller

Class of 1927
Helen French Stuter
Helen Irwin
Wilhelmina Ross May
Hazel Smith Port
Romaine Gorsuch Conrad
Florence Penrod Walker
Laura Sensor Patterson
Hazel Whitsel Meloy

Class of 1928
Ruth Jones
Thelma Hoover Johnston
Ruth Esther McMillin Lynn
Louise Freeberg Stever
Helen Isenberg
Helen McNeel Morrow
Ina Wright LaRue
Margaret Gearinger Van Loan
Veronica Brennan
Kathryn Brennen Snyder
Alma Freberg Barto

Class of 1929
Pearl Houtz
Fleeta Foor Layton
Maude Morningstar Brett
Esther Rath Walkey
Mary Kegg Beegle
Gertrude Preston
Pauline Treaster

Class of 1930
Edith Abbott Brandt
Evalyn Baughman McClay
Gladys Brown Seager
Helen Irwin Miller
Jeanette Showalter Mench
Pauline Wallace Wallace

Class of 1931
Irene Neider Erbe
Martha Huff Harvey
Edna Park
Nellie McIntyre Leighty
Norma Baker
Sara Donelson Dudek
Mabel Wolfe Price
Mary Crum Fields
Martha Hickes Smith
Marguerite Bales Bennett
Helen Oberlander Woods
Helena Mierley Werner

Class of 1932
Evelyn Mairs Davidson
Hazel Rhodes Orner
Gladys Abbott Badman
Harriet Robb
Betty Welch Solomon
Doris Pennell Megahan
Romaine Kegg Hershberger
Theo Welch Santocrose
Louise Weaver Beaver
Vernetta Bumgardner

Class of 1933
Catherine McIlroy Karns
Mary Kephart Bayer
Nancy Strausser
Mary Patterson
Mary Madden Hautman
Ada Deffibaugh Heffner
Suie Deffibaugh Mateer

Class of 1934
Erma Brown Parsons
Catherine Whitsel
Emma Foor Pick
Mary Halbbaugh Wilson
Jean Galbraith Bollinger
Clementine Zeigler Asper
Althea Cupp Cleck
Ruby Patton Cook
Violet Baughman Saylor
Jeanette Anderson Schell
Jane Walton McKeon

Class of 1935
Josephine Filson Corbin
Alma Defibaugh Rupert
Ruth Keith Prendergast
Gertrude Lane Gutshall
Esther Reihart Coffman
Laura Isenberg White
Mary Hefsel Bowers
Dorothy Rutter Adams
Elizabeth Prendergast Stallings
Clara Koontz Black
Janie Winter Crouse

Class of 1936
Pauline Adams Bollinger
Winifred Bair Dougherty
Anna Briggs Fowler
Emma Fouse Pidcock
Margaret Thompson Hutchison

Class of 1937
Beatrice Brumbaugh Port
Ivy Burns Krider
Mary Gutshall Miller
Elizabeth Hitchens Shenefelt
Josephine Keith Davis
Phyllis Moreland Hall
Charlotte Shaw Myers
Electa Felton Mears

Class of 1938
Lena Carbaugh Clapper
Martha Cavender Platt
Velva Dick
Carolyn Guyer Honsacker
Margery Metz Duncan
Martha Keith Laester
Mary Mayes Showalter
Leona Park Price
Virginia Snyder Guyer
Edna Williams Albright

Class of 1939
Eleanor Blough Kimmel
Ethel Brumbaugh
Mary Frederick Dick
Esther Lewis Meloy
Doris Porter Thompson
Lucille Weiser Shultz
Ruth Weaver Yama
Daphne Weston Linderberger
Edna Worthing Wertman

Class of 1940
Evelyn Knittle Temple
Jean Metz Stone
Virginia Bollman Filiatreault
Dorothy Kemp MacNamara
Grace Hile DeLong
Valeria Struble Wible
Mary Myers
Mary Shunp
Dorothy Pearce McFarland

In Training When
School Closed
Althea Hallibaugh Weyant
Lillian Carlson Stevens
Lucille Anderson
Dorothy Hendrick Underhill
Pearl Confer Nembauer

PRESENTED BY THE AUXILIARY TO J.C. BLAIR MEMORIAL HOSPITAL 2009

As a centennial project, the Auxiliary replaced a damaged plaque that was originally dedicated in 1974 to the graduates of the J. C. Blair Memorial Hospital School of Nursing. The new plaque, dedicated November 2, 2009, honors the 186 nurses who received diplomas from the school.

48

Four

NURSES TRAINING SCHOOL

Just three months after J. C. Blair Memorial Hospital opened its doors, it launched a three-year nurses' training program. Brochures promised prospective students that earning a diploma would net them the "substantial personal profit" of at least $25 a week.

Interest in this opportunity ran so high that two classes graduated from the school in 1915, the first—the class of 1914—on February 12 and the second group on November 19. Sixteen additional young women were in training, and a nurses' residence, with room for 30 students, had risen up beside the hospital.

Plans for the hospital had always included a nursing school. Speaking on Physicians' and Press Day, Dr. Francis P. Ball declared, "The advent of the trained nurse, the direct product of the modern hospital, has been one of the greatest boons to the sick." Dr. Theodore L. Chase added: "For the girl who desires to enter a professional career, there is not a field open to women which presents a better opportunity for inspired and distinguished service to her fellow-beings than that of the graduate nurse."

Twenty-seven classes of registered nurses graduated before changes in state requirements closed the school in 1940. Nine nurses graduated that year; five remaining students transferred elsewhere to complete their training. J. C. Blair Memorial Hospital's school graduated 186 nurses, who scattered far and wide. But no matter how far they traveled, these women never forgot their nursing school years, when their shared experiences forged friendships that endured for the rest of their lives.

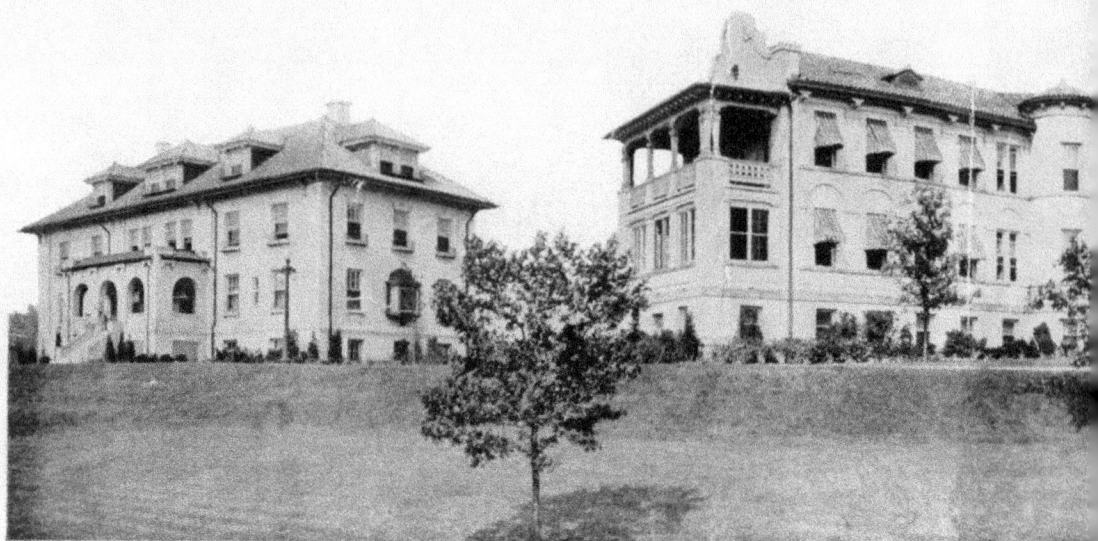

NURSES HOME—1916

Nurses Training School

J. C. Blair Memorial Hospital

❖ ❖ ❖ ❖ ❖

YOUNG LADIES

WE INVITE your earnest attention to a career of splendid service to the public and substantial personal profit. Nursing shares with the practice of medicine in being the noblest profession in the world. Never at the beck and call of a boss, you are your own master. Sources of employment are never lacking. There is always a tremendous call for you. In general work you make $25.00 or more a week and in institutional work from $60.00 to $150.00 per month. In addition to this, no other business open to women promises such an avenue of social advancement.

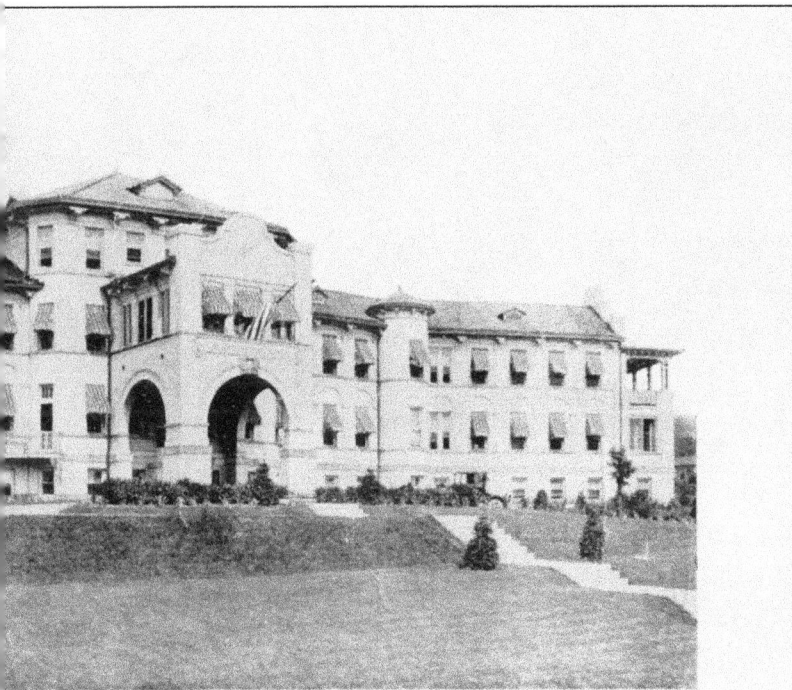
MEMORIAL HOSPITAL—1911

C. Blair Memorial Hospital offers a thoroughly equip-
g school. All living expenses are paid in one of the
itful nurses' homes in Pennsylvania and a liberal allow-
•ney, after the first three months of the probationary
complete course of lectures, approved by the Pennsyl-
d of Registration for Nurses.

cept pupils with one or more years of high school
its educational equivalent.

or an application blank and in three years be a fully
id equipped trained nurse.

ss Miss P. Schneider, Supt., Huntingdon, Pa.

How many young women must have read this brochure with eagerness and hope? Each one fortunate enough to have her application approved would need to pass a physical exam before beginning her training. Following a two-month probation period, if she qualified, she would officially become a student nurse. Three years of hard work lay ahead of her.

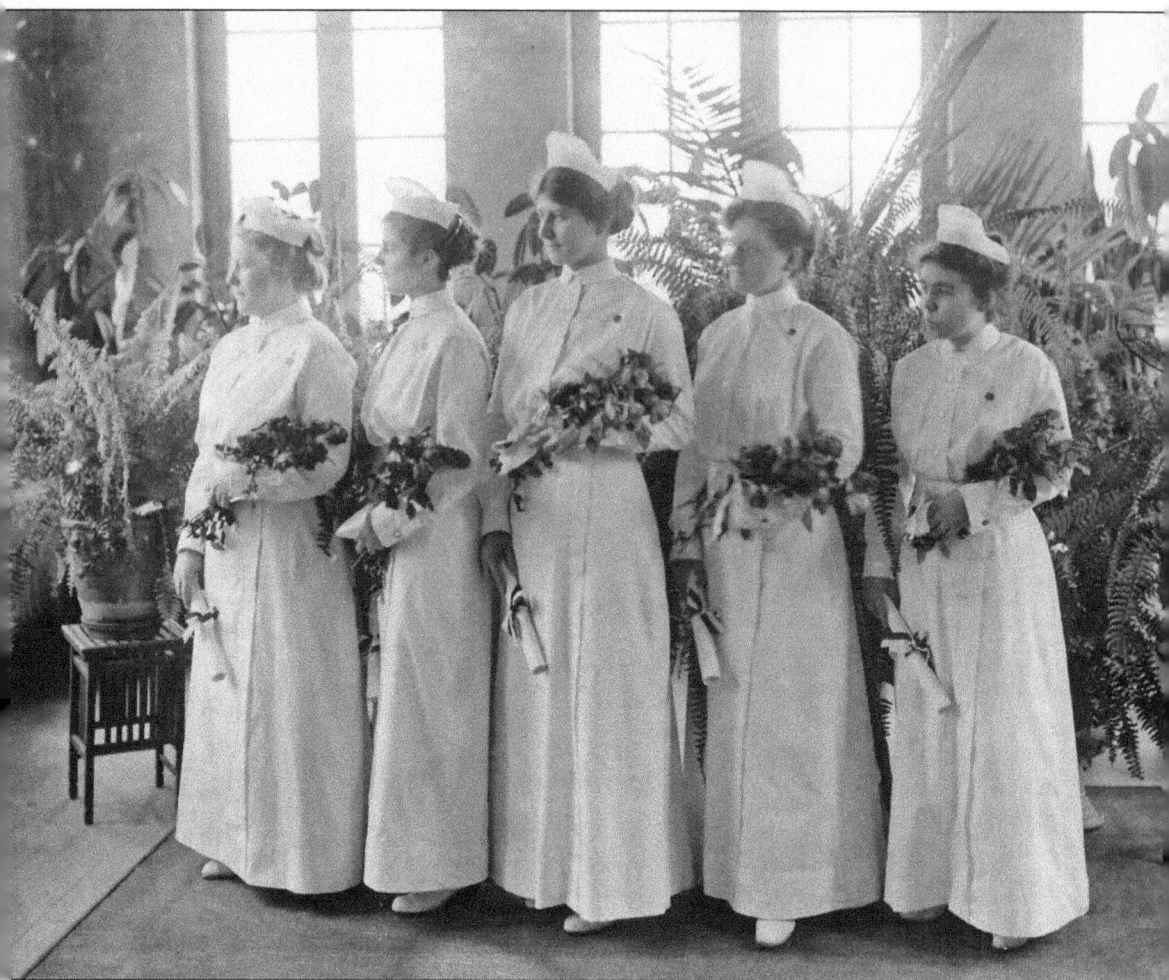

The Nurses Training School opened on December 4, 1911, with a class of six. All but one young woman completed the three-year course and graduated on February 12, 1915. Dr. Francis P. Ball, former president of the Pennsylvania Medical Society, delivered the address; Professor I. Harvey Brumbaugh, president of Juniata College, presented the diplomas; and Dr. H. C. Frontz, chairman of the Training School Committee, presented the class pins. The class of 1914 photograph shows the proud graduates. From left to right are Lida McAfee Leonard, Port Royal, Juniata County; Lucy Hamilton Coughton, Cassville; Anna Rachel Garner, Marklesburg; Elsie Grace Lightner, Huntingdon; and Blanche Isenberg Parks, Alexandria. During World War I, Leonard served in the Army Nurse Corps and Garner served with the American Red Cross.

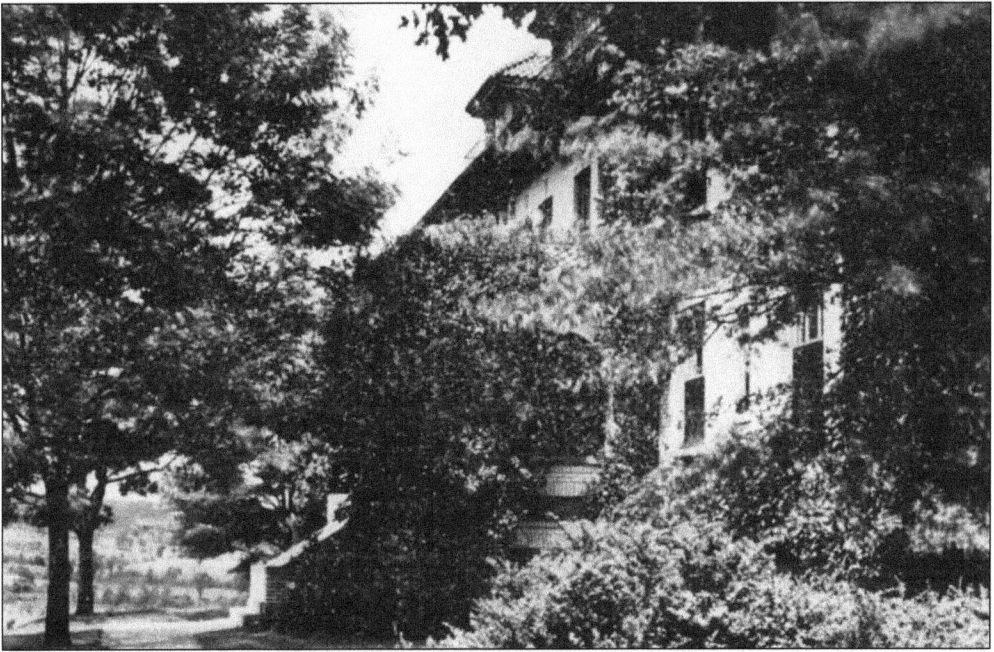

In 1912, Kate Fisher Blair offered to erect a building to house the student nurses. Four years later, the Nurses' Home opened with rooms for 30 nurses. Leafy trees shaded the building on pleasant days. For cold weather, nurses were advised to bring a wrap to wear between the home and the hospital.

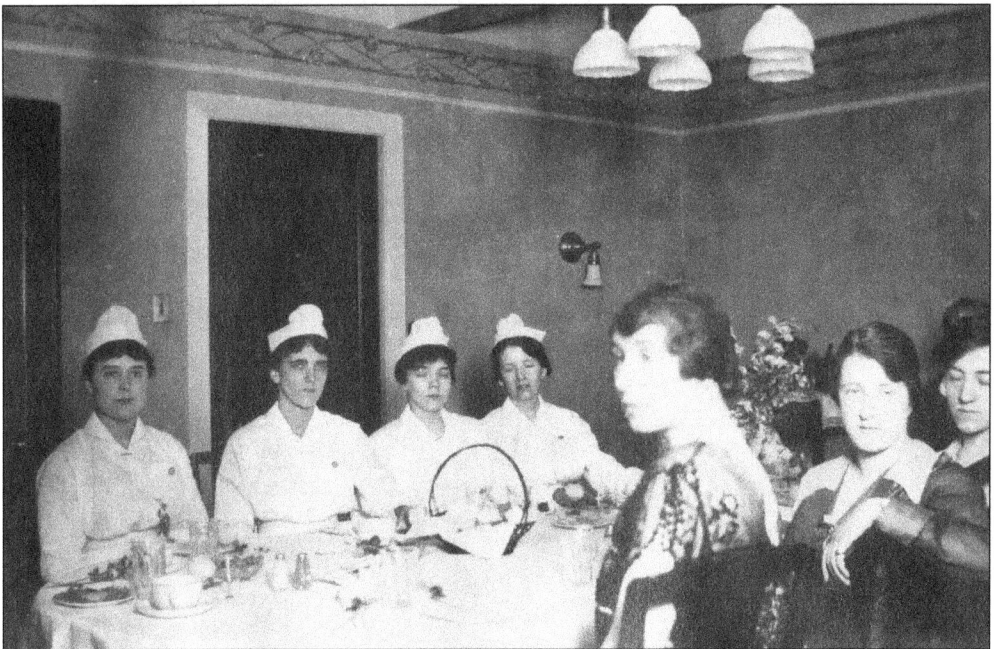

Beginning at 6:30 each morning, the nurses began arriving in the dining room for breakfast. Dinner was served from noon until 1:00 p.m. and supper between 5:00 and 6:00 each evening. Each nurse was to provide her own napkin ring. Punctual attendance at meals was required, and students would need special permission to miss one.

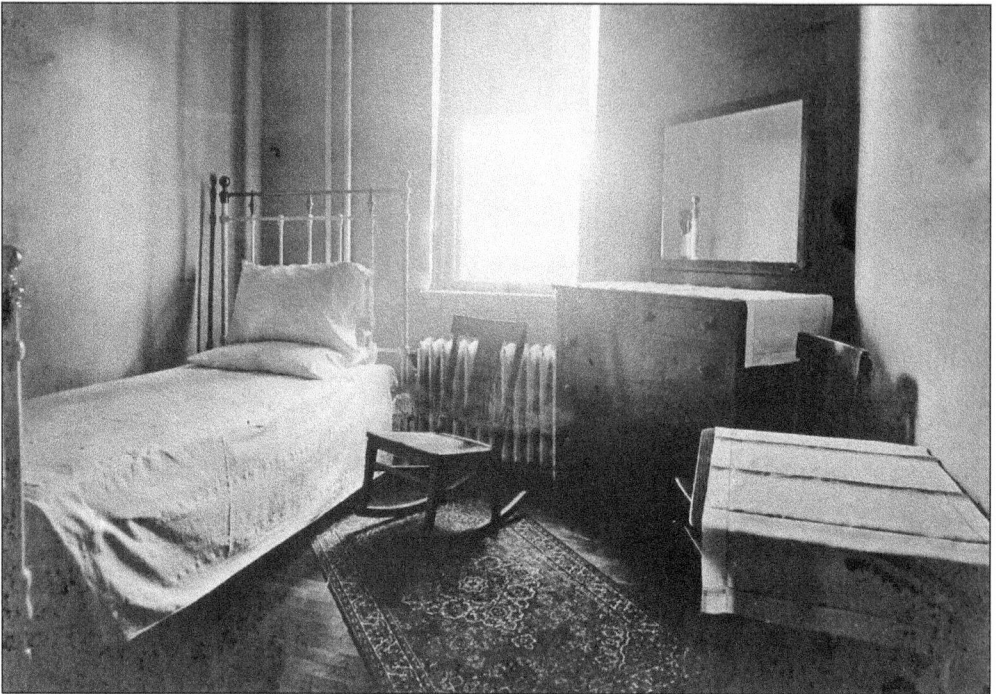

Nurses' Home rules recommended that a student attend three meals and get eight hours of sleep each night. She was to bring a pair of black oxfords with rubber heels, six pairs of black stockings, two plain wash dresses, one pair of overshoes or galoshes, and "plenty of plain underwear well marked with indelible ink or nametape." She was required to have her room in "such condition that it may be inspected at any time." The small, private rooms were strictly utilitarian in design, with sparse furnishings taking up most of the space. Still, there was room for fun, such as this Saint Patrick's Day party. (Both, courtesy of Thomas F. Miller.)

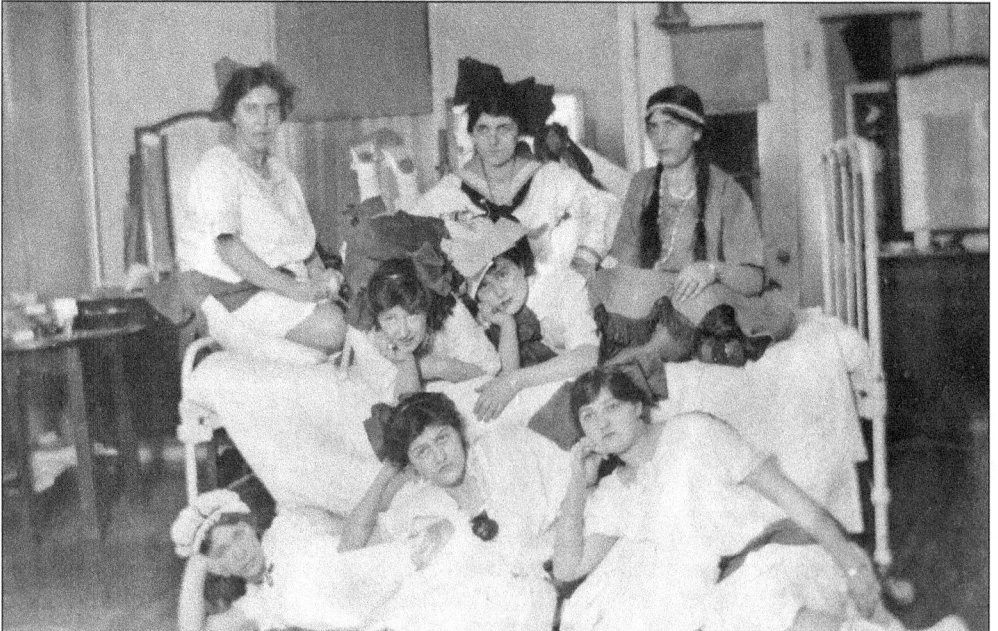

When Gladys Zerbe Miller (class of 1918) was a student, Anna Rachel Garner (class of 1914) was on the staff at the hospital. She had worked as a nurse at J. C. Blair before attaining the position of supervisor. Gladys snapped this photograph of her at the rear of the Nurses' Home. (Courtesy of Thomas F. Miller.)

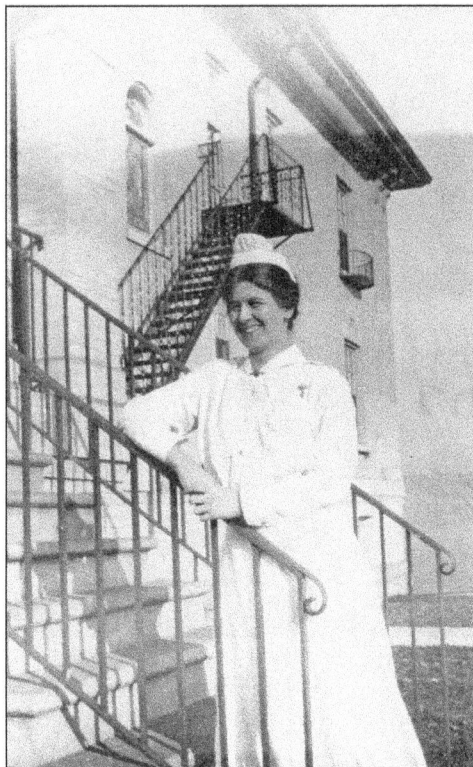

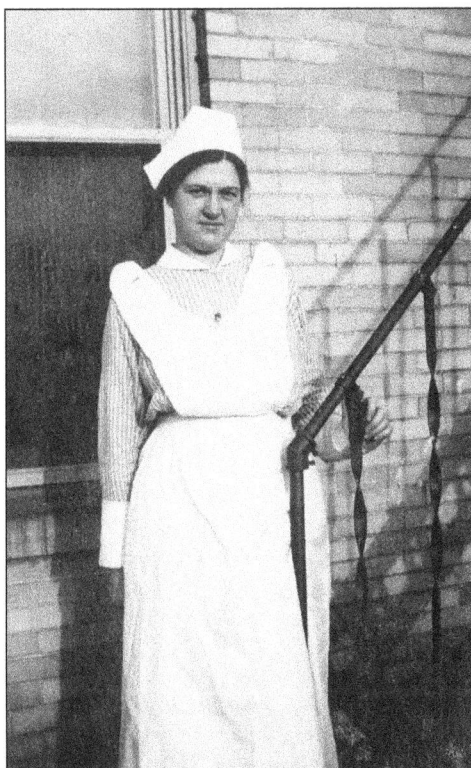

The dress code required student nurses to wear uniforms in the hospital but not to wear them beyond hospital property. The hospital provided one uniform; each student had to purchase 2 more dresses and 10 aprons. (Courtesy of Thomas F. Miller.)

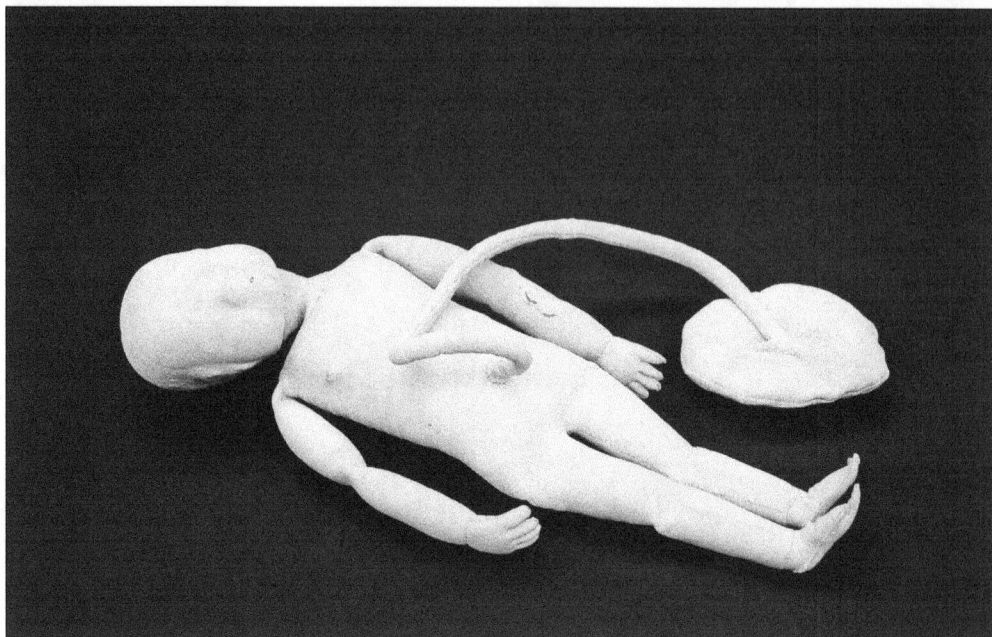

This leather doll served as a teaching aid. Olive M. Bayer, training school instructor, taught the functions of reproductive organs to first-year students. The following year, Dr. Cloy G. Brumbaugh lectured on pregnancy and finished the final year with sessions on obstetrics. (Photograph by Linda Cutshall.)

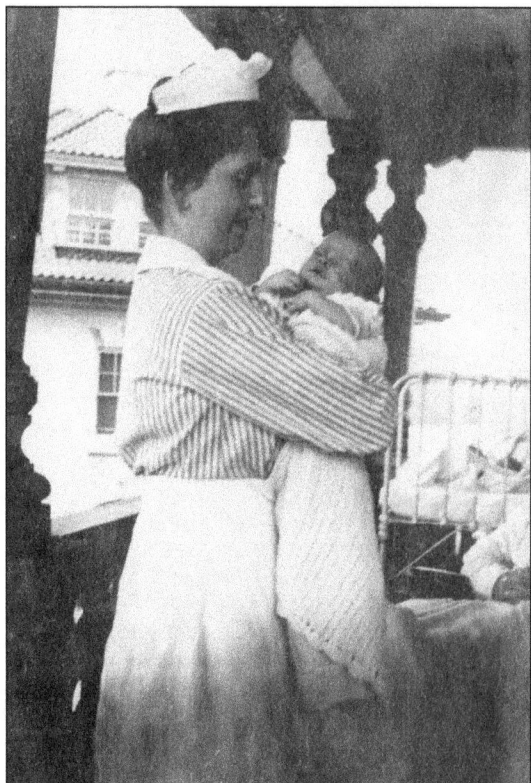

Fae Painter Brown, class of 1917, held this real, live baby on one of the hospital's airy porches. Second and third year students studied diseases and "artificial feeding" of infants, followed by the general care of the youngest patients. Dr. G. G. Harman and Dr. Brumbaugh were instructors on these subjects. (Courtesy of Thomas F. Miller.)

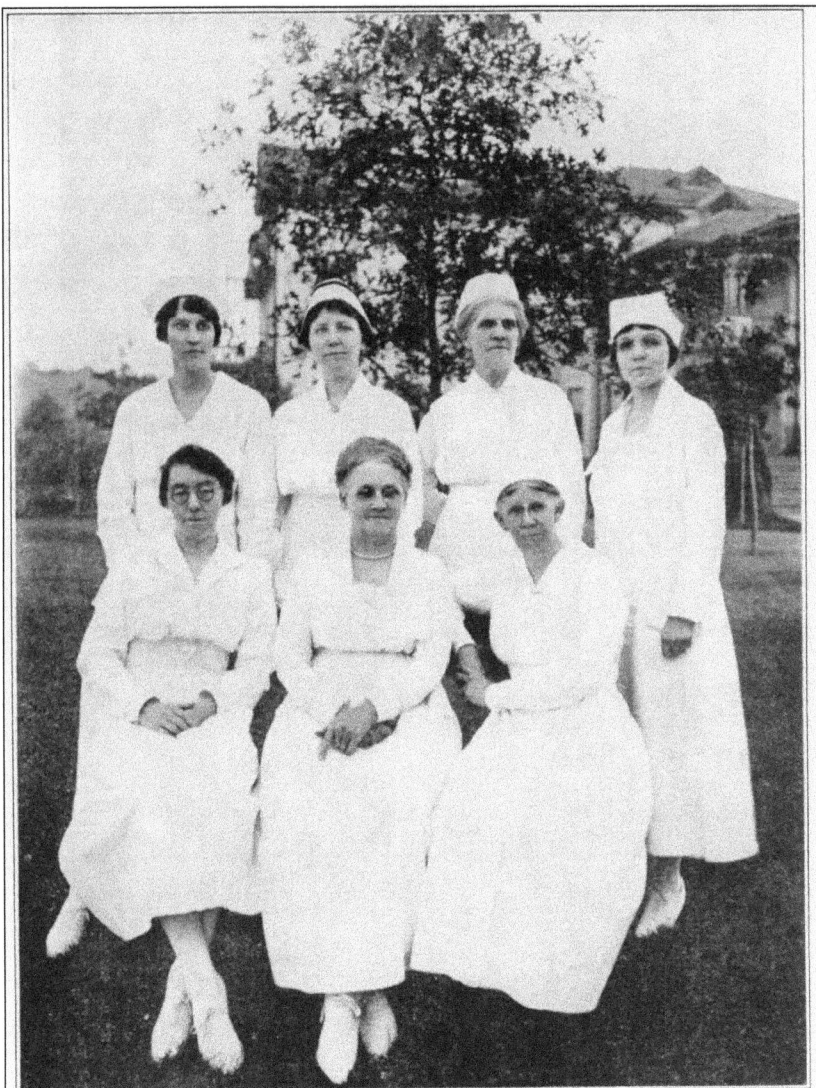

Faculty

MISS PENA SCHNEIDER, R. N, Superintendent.
MISS OLIVE M. BAYER, R. N, Instructress of Training School.
MISS BERNICE McKEE, R. N, Floor Supervisor.
MISS GRETTA WESTON, R. N, Operating Room Supervisor.
MISS DOROTHY RUNG, R. N, Night Supervisor.
MISS VERNICE GELVIN, Dietician.
MRS. ELLA MILLER, Matron of Nurses' Home.

Given the positions listed after their names, it appears that the heading of "faculty" may be misleading; only one of the women pictured filled a faculty position in the Nurses Training School. A 1919–1920 brochure, giving a complete list of courses required in the three-year program, identifies Drs. Frontz, Sears, Chisolm, Harman, Schum, Fetterhoof, Brumbaugh, and Hutchison as the nursing school instructors. In addition, Olive Bayer taught three courses to first-year students. The image comes from *The Book of the Nine*, the class of 1922 yearbook. The class was the largest in the school's history, up to that time, and the young women adopted the nickname of "The Nine," which is reflected in their yearbook's title.

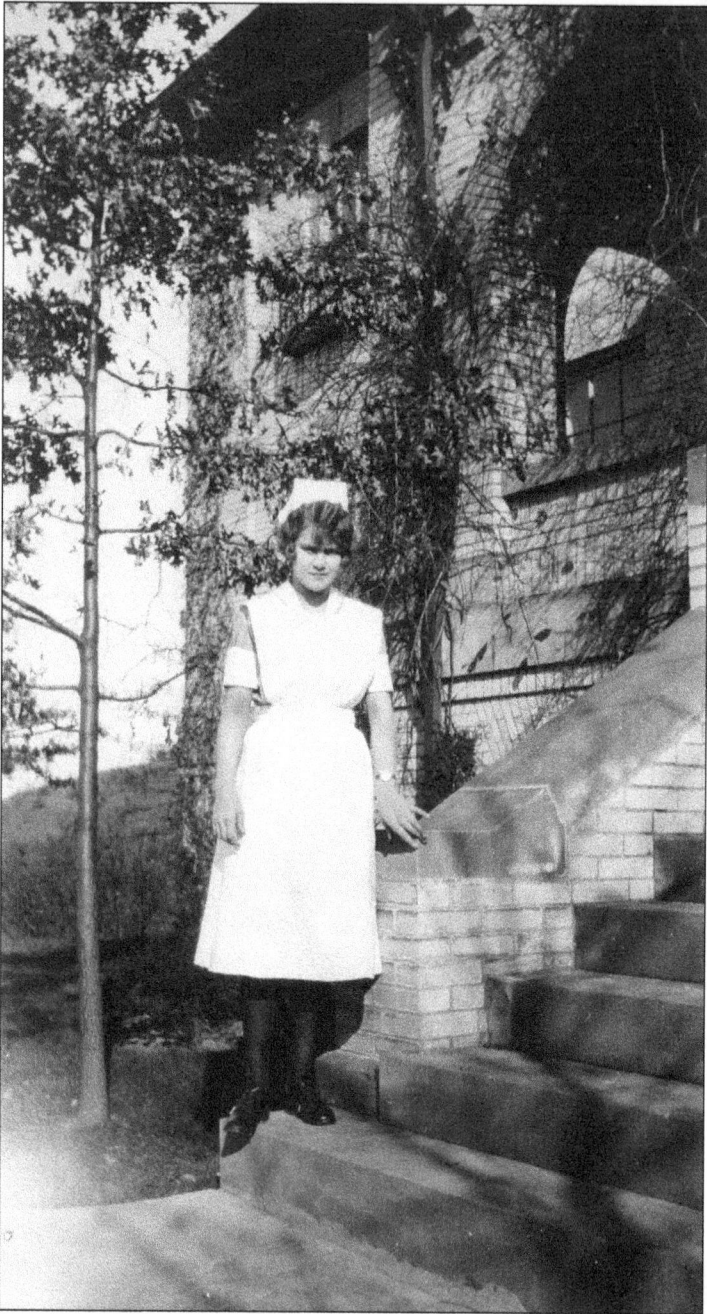

Sporting her white nurse's cap, Gladys Brown Seager, class of 1930, posed on the steps of the Nurses' Home. Gladys wore a long, white "pinny" or pinafore over her short-sleeved uniform. The dress code for student nurses also required black stockings and shoes. On her left wrist she wore a watch—one with a second hand, as required by the school. Board, lodging, laundry, and medical care were free, with a monthly allowance ($10 the first year, $12.50 the second, and $15 the third) to pay for uniforms and textbooks. Each year, she could look forward to two vacations with pay: two weeks in the summer, one week in the winter, plus 10 days of sick leave if needed, during her training.

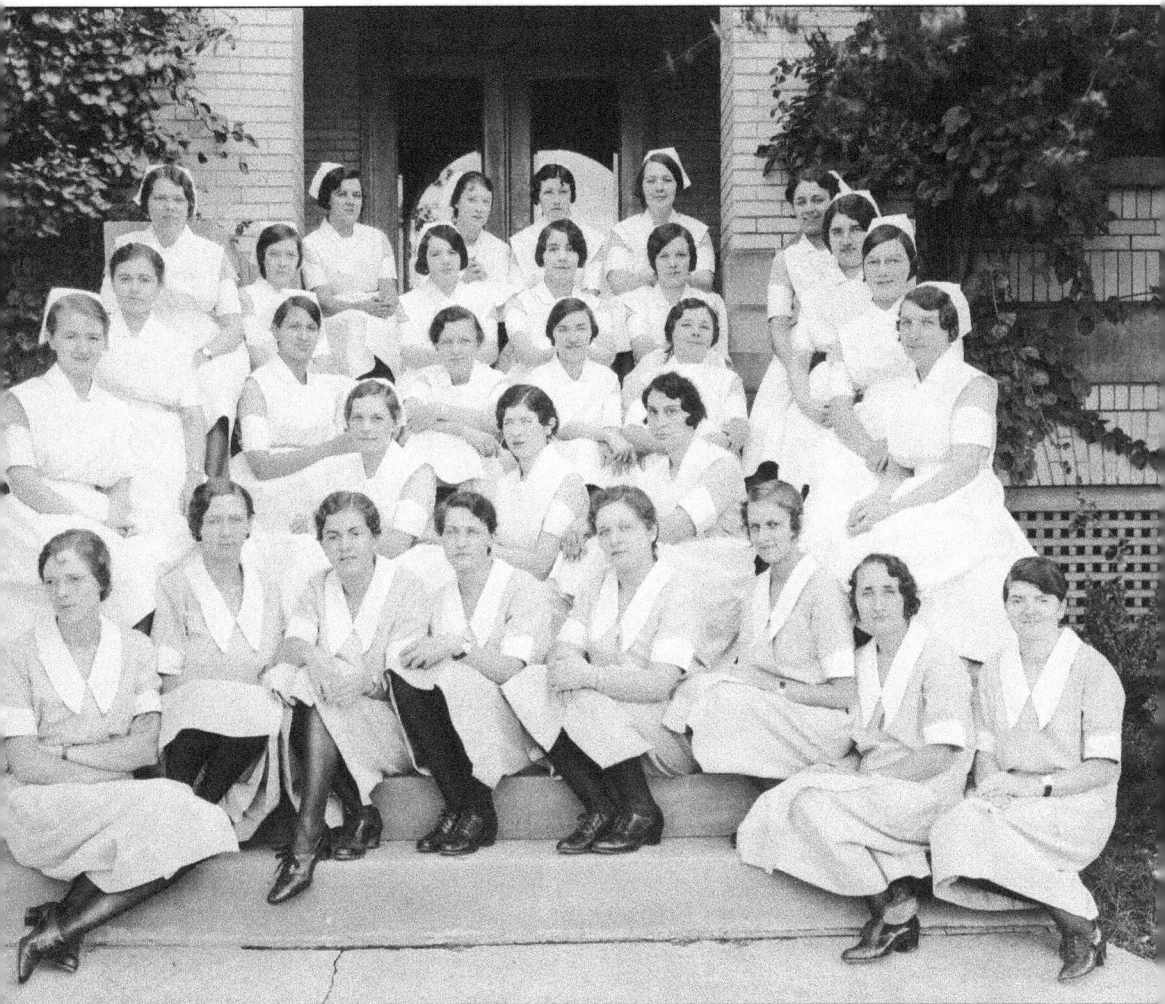

Members of the classes of 1931 through 1934 gathered for a photograph on the steps of the Nurses' Home. Catherine McIlroy Karns, class of 1933, identified these members of the group: Clementine Zeigler Asper, Jean Galbraith Bollinger, Jeannette Anderson Schell, Erma Brown Parsons, Marguerite Bales Bennett, Martha Hickes Smith, Mabel Wolfe Price, Suie Deffibaugh Mateer, Mary Madden Haulman, Catherine Whitsel, Catherine McIlroy Karns, Mary Kephart Bayer, Nancy Strauser, Mary Hallibaugh Wilson, Mary Patterson, Ada Deffibaugh Heffner, Nancy Foor Pick, Gladys Abbott Badman, Louise Weaver Beaver, Harriet Robb, and Doris Pennel Megahan. Note the different uniforms they wore; the "prebies," or probationary students (first row), have distinctly different uniforms. (Courtesy of Marcelene Karns Baker.)

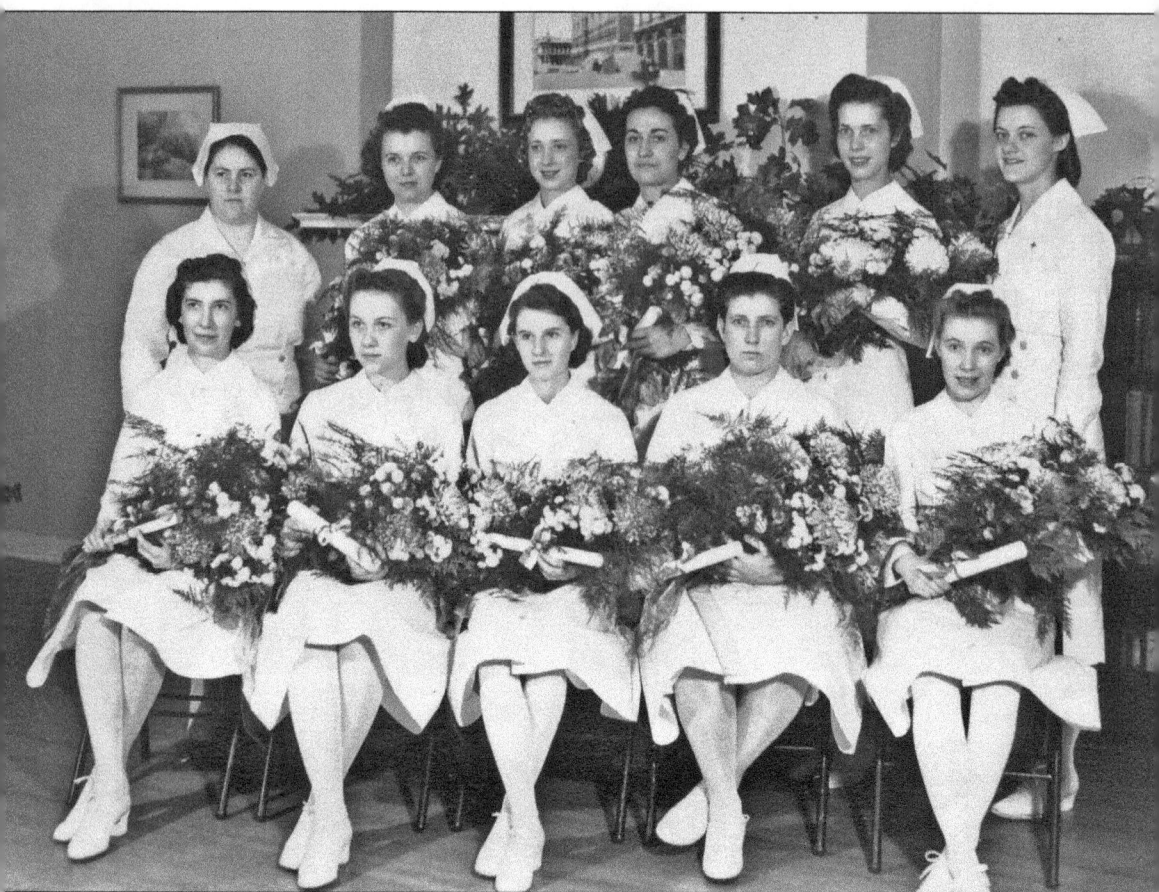

In 1940, J. C. Blair Memorial Hospital's Nurses Training School graduated its last class. Posing for the photographer are, from left to right, (first row) Dorothy Kemp MacNamara, Huntingdon; Grace Hile DeLong, Saxton; Dorothy Pearce McFarland, Penns Grove, New Jersey; and Mary Shimp and Valeria Struble Wible, State College; (second row) Nettie Bealer, instructor; Jean Metz Stone, Waterstreet; Mary Myers Elder, State College; Evelyn Knittle Temple, Shamokin; Virginia Bollman Filiatreault, Defiance; and the unidentified assistant instructor. Five students in training when the school closed—Althea Hallibaugh Weyant, Lillian Carlson Stevens, Lucille Anderson, Dorothy Hendrick Underhill, and Pearl Confer Nembauer—finished their degrees at Montgomery Hospital in Norristown. (Courtesy of Virginia Filiatreault.)

J. C. Blair graduates served at home and abroad during wartime. During World War I, Anna Rachel Garner (1914) and Mildred Neff (1916) worked for the American Red Cross. Lida McAfee Leonard (1914) and Gladys Zerbe Miller (1918) joined the Army Nurse Corps. This photograph shows Miller (wearing her cape) at Camp Sevier in Greenville, South Carolina. (Courtesy of Thomas F. Miller.)

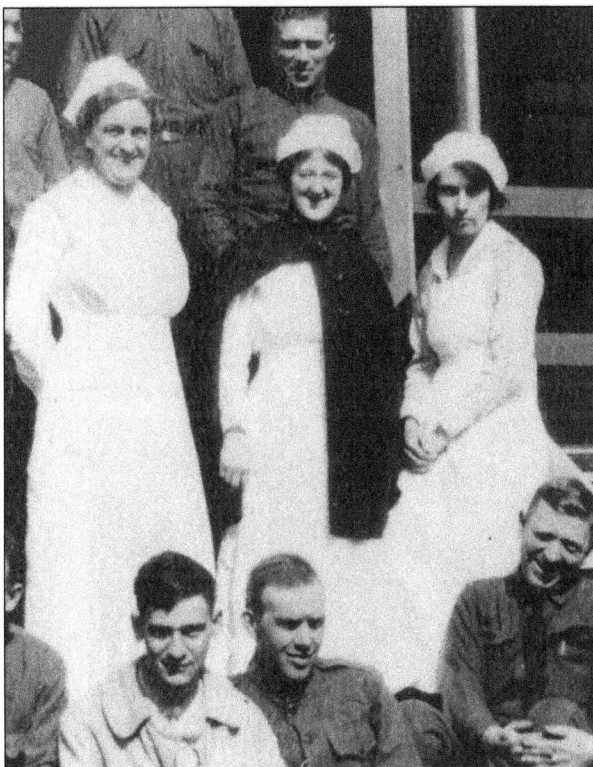

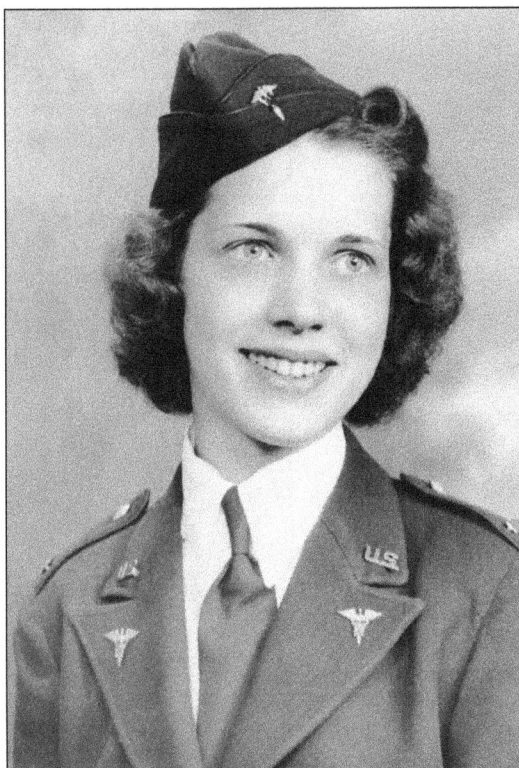

Nine graduates served in World War II: Maj. Veronica Brennan (1928), Lt. Col. Edna Park (1931), Lt. Col. Mary Patterson (1933), Lt. Dorothy Rutter Adams (1935), 1st Lt. Marjorie Metz Duncan (1938), Lt. Ethel Brumbaugh (1939), Lt. Mary Myers (1940), 1st Lt. Jean Metz Stone (1940), and Lt. Virginia Bollman Filiatreault (1940), pictured. Virginia met her husband in Italy and was married wearing a gown she made herself of parachute silk. (Courtesy of Virginia Filiatreault.)

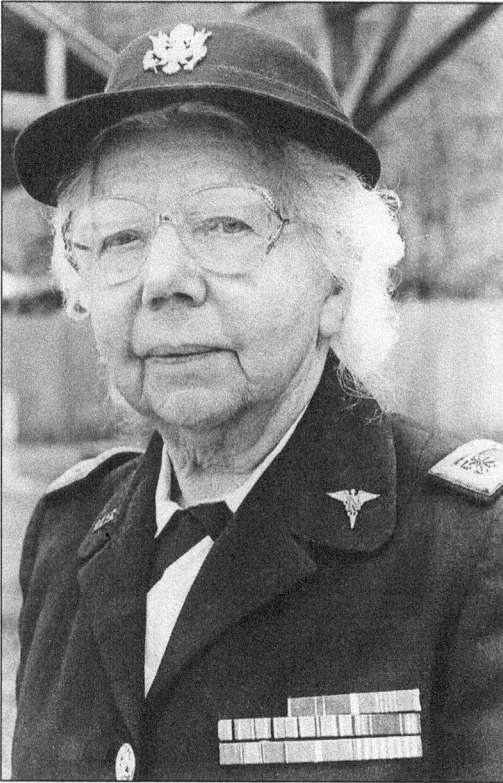

Edna Park enlisted in the Army Nurse Corps in 1941, about 10 years after graduating from nursing school. She was first assigned to the 181st Military General Hospital in India; later, during the Korean War, she was the command nurse in a Mobile Army Surgical Hospital (MASH) unit. She went on to log more than 18 years of army service. A native of Saxton, she was a familiar figure in local Memorial Day and Veterans Day parades after her retirement, as seen here. (Courtesy of Ron Morgan.)

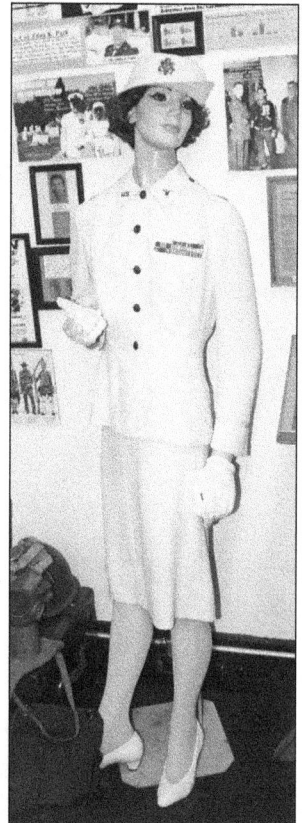

One of Park's uniforms is exhibited at the Broad Top Area Coal Miners Museum in Robertsdale, where many aspects of Broad Top area history are on display. Park earned nine medals during her military service, including the Bronze Star, the World War II Victory Medal, the Asiatic-Pacific Campaign Medal, and the Korean Service Medal. (Courtesy of Ron Morgan.)

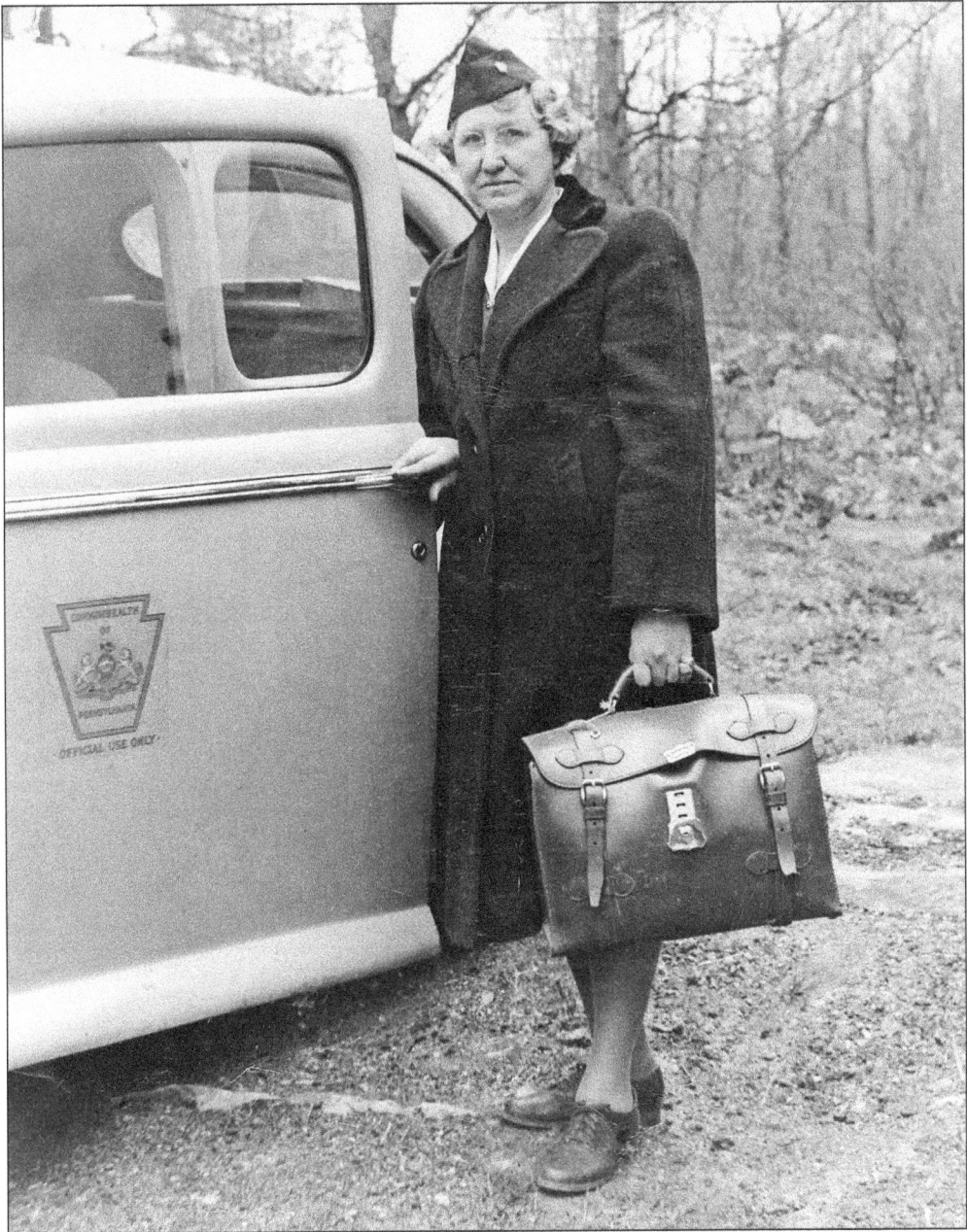

Public health nurses take their skills directly to people in need of health information and medical attention. Pearl Hamilton, class of 1925, was a public health nurse for almost 30 years. Other graduates who followed the same career included Thelma Showalter Miller (1925), Kathryn Brennen Snyder (1928), Marguerite Bales Bennett (1931), Janie Winter Crouse (1935), and Althea Hallibaugh Weyant, a student when the school closed. (Courtesy of Jon Baughman.)

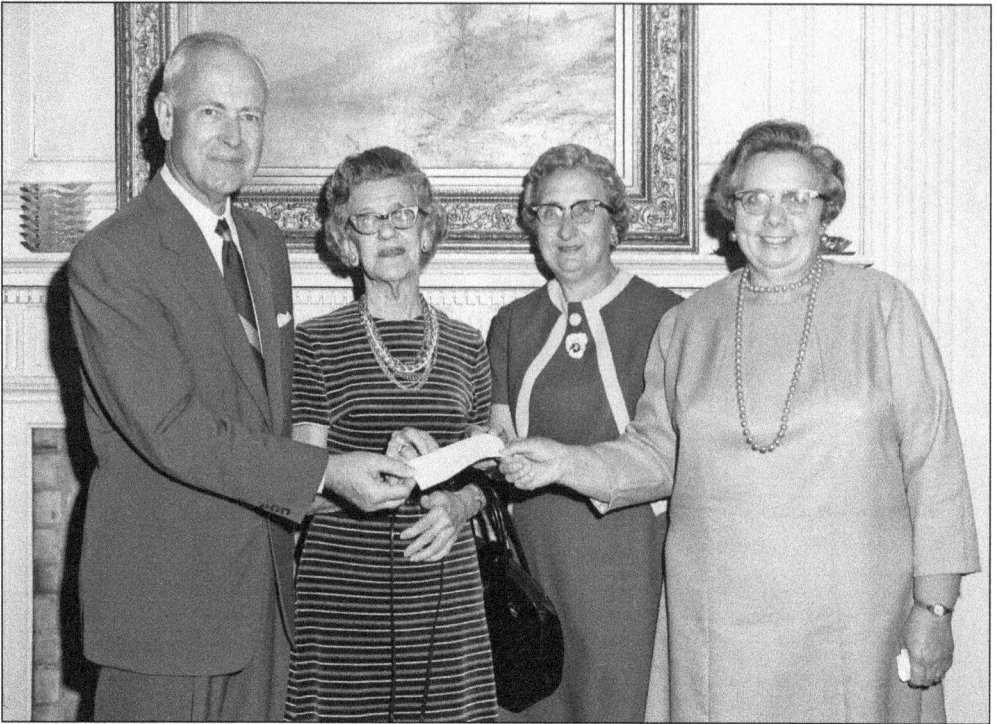

The Nurses' Alumnae Association helped J. C. Blair graduates maintain their affectionate ties with each other and with the hospital. In 1970, Julia Craig (1920), Jeannette Schell (1934), and Mary Showalter (1938)—all lifelong employees of Blair Hospital, as well as graduates of its nursing school—presented John A. Kunz, campaign chairman, with $500 for the Acute Care Wing building fund. At about the same time, the alumnae saved the name and cartouche from the 1911 building's front entrance when it was replaced by a modern covered drive-through. The salvaged elements were incorporated into a low wall facing Bryan Street. Later they became important elements in the new entrance created for the 1950 building. (See page 98.)

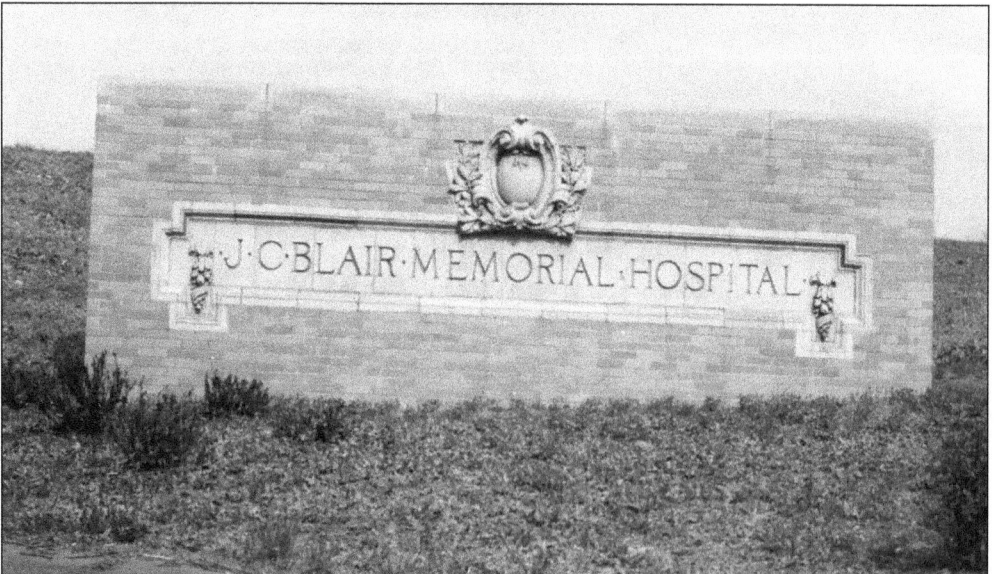

Five

DOCTORS

J. C. Blair Memorial Hospital was blessed from its beginning with a staff of doctors who strongly supported its development and who willingly did double duty as instructors in its nurses training program. Through the efforts of these doctors, and of the Board of Trustees and the Ladies Auxiliary, the institution saw increasing acceptance and use of its facilities, greater community support, and more physicians drawn to practice in the surrounding area.

Certification in specialized fields of medicine is a relatively recent development in the profession, but J. C. Blair Memorial Hospital, from the beginning, designated staff positions in surgery, medicine, and x-ray. Members of the small, early staff might, out of necessity, have more than one field of responsibility. But within the first decade of its existence, the hospital had enough staff with a variety of interests and knowledge to fill the specialized positions with doctors who had concentrated on an area of study and pursued advanced training and experience.

Throughout the hospital's century of service, the institution has been successful in attracting— sometimes by chance, sometimes by recruitment—a corps of physicians capable of treating the varied medical conditions that patients experience. Replacement of retiring doctors is somewhat generational: an influx occurred in the 1930s and 1940s to replace the earlier staff, and again in the 1970s, a generational shift occurred. Those doctors are now beginning to retire, and another recruitment effort is ongoing.

Present at the births, illnesses, and deaths of those they care for, doctors have unusually intimate relationships with their patients, offering support and counsel in time of stress. Thus, many doctors affiliated with J. C. Blair Memorial Hospital through the years have earned the respect, and even love, of the communities they serve.

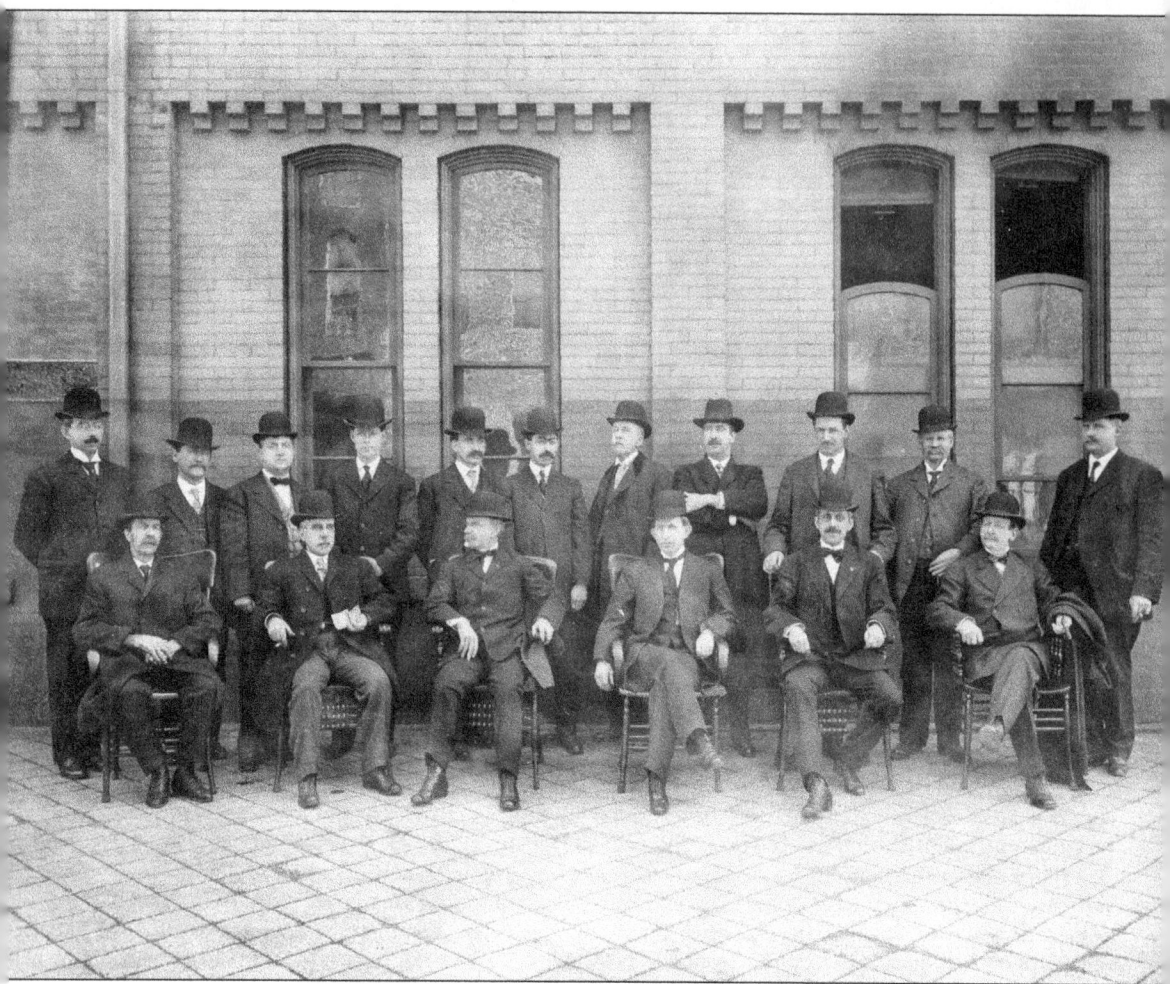

The Huntingdon County Medical Society gathered at the railroad station for this group portrait in 1908, just three years before the opening of J. C. Blair Memorial Hospital. They are identified as, from left to right, (first row) Dr. M. R. Evans, Huntingdon; Dr. George G. Harman, Huntingdon; Dr. Charles B. Bush, Orbisonia; Dr. Robert H. Moore, Huntingdon; Dr. Howard C. Frontz, Huntingdon; and Dr. George W. Simpson, Mill Creek; (second row) Dr. William H. Sears, Huntingdon; Dr. William J. Campbell, Mount Union; Dr. John M. Steel, Huntingdon; Dr. John B. Beck, Alexandria; Dr. C. A. R. McClain, Mount Union; Dr. Landon; Dr. Alvin R. McCarthy, Mount Union; Dr. William H. Boggs, Huntingdon; Dr. John C. Stever, Mount Union; Dr. John C. Fleming, Shirleysburg; and Dr. J. M. Johnston, Huntingdon. Drs. Frontz, Harman, Steel, and Sears were on the staff of the hospital when it opened, while Drs. Beck, Simpson, McClain, Campbell, and Bush—with practices located some distance from the hospital—were on the consulting staff.

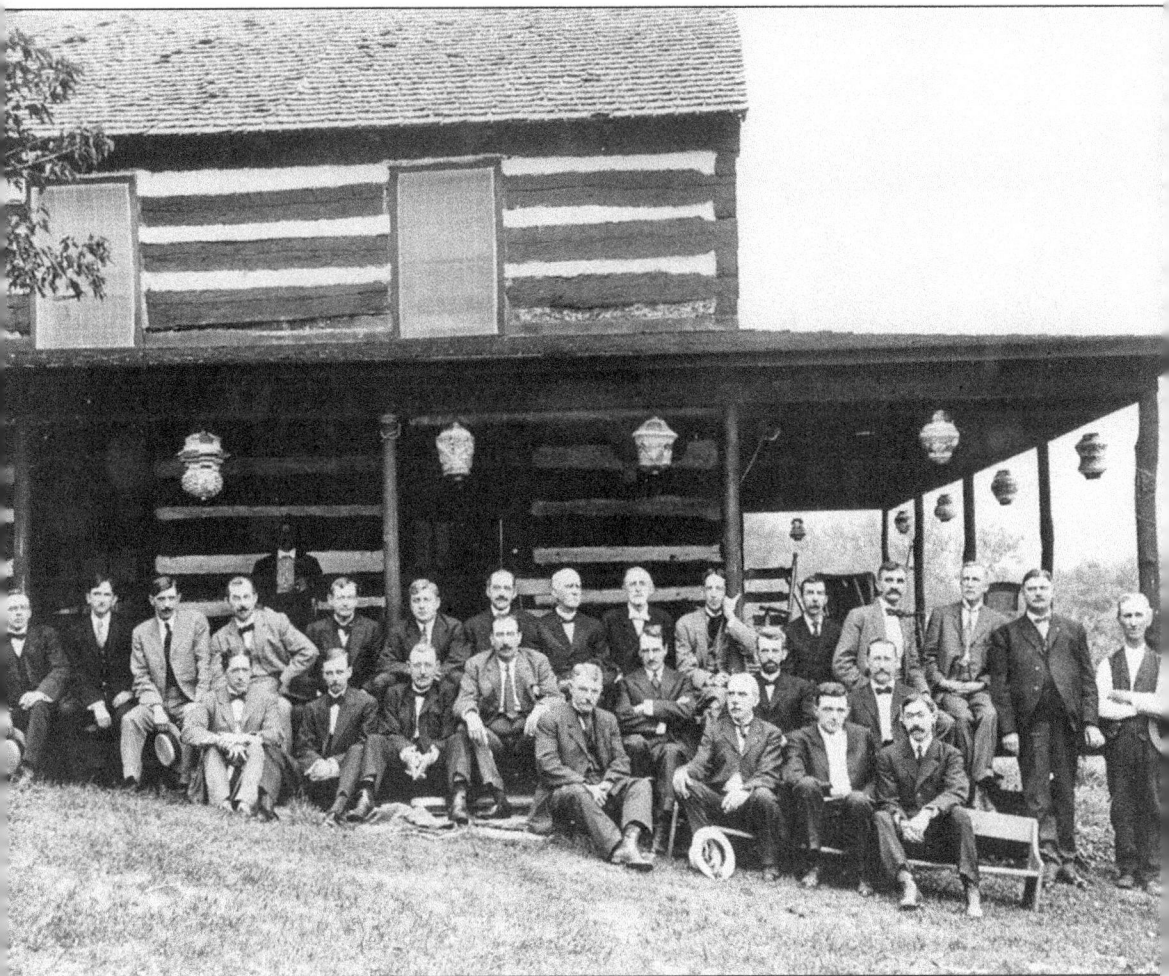

The Huntingdon County Medical Society also enjoyed more casual pursuits, such as this outing, also in 1908, at pharmacist Harry Read's summer cottage on the Raystown Branch. But casual dress was not much different from their more formal attire seen on the opposite page. Straw boaters replaced felt bowlers, however, as the headgear of choice for summer. Not all in this group are identified, but those that are include five not seen in the railroad station image: Drs. Keichline, Brumbaugh, Carney, Myers, and Miller. Pictured are (first row) Harry Read, Dr. Harman, and two unidentified; (second row) Dr. Beck, Dr. John M. Keichline, Petersburg; unidentified; Dr. Boggs; Dr. Stever, and two unidentified; (third row) Dr. Cloy G. Brumbaugh, Huntingdon; Dr. Joseph A. Carney, Robertsdale; unidentified; Dr. Sears; two unidentified; Dr. Frontz; Dr. Rudolph Myers, Huntingdon; Dr. David P. Miller, Huntingdon; Dr. Moore; Dr. Evans; two unidentified; Dr. Johnston; and one unidentified.

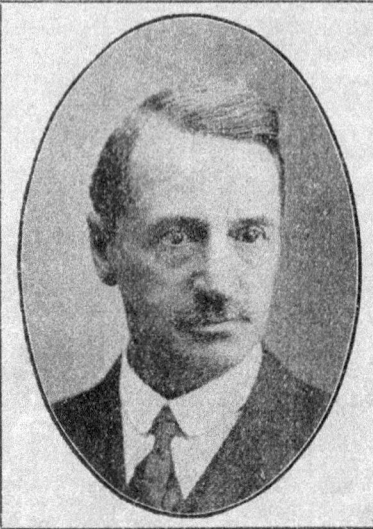

DR. STEVER

Offices opposite E. B. T. R. R. Depot

MOUNT UNION, - PA.

Hours: 8 a. m. to 8 p. m.   Phone·

Sundays by Appointment.

I am a regular office specialist. I treat all the ills of the human body. My offices are equipped with all of the modern instruments of precision. The fee is fifty cents in cash, medicine included.

I do a large amount of eye, ear, nose and throat work, including the fitting of glasses, satisfaction guaranteed. My charges are reasonable and the fees are always agreed upon beforehand.

Acute and Chronic diseases treated with the Hot Air Body Apparatus, such as rheumatism, diseases of the joints, swellings and painful maladies.

Ailments peculiar to the sexes are treated in the strictest privacy. Rupture cured by the injection method without operation.

Consultation by Mail

Mail orders promptly filled for the home cure of the drink habit and bed wetting of children. If you wish to consult me by letter enclose $1.00, (currency will do) and write me full particulars. I will supply the medicine.

Address your letters:

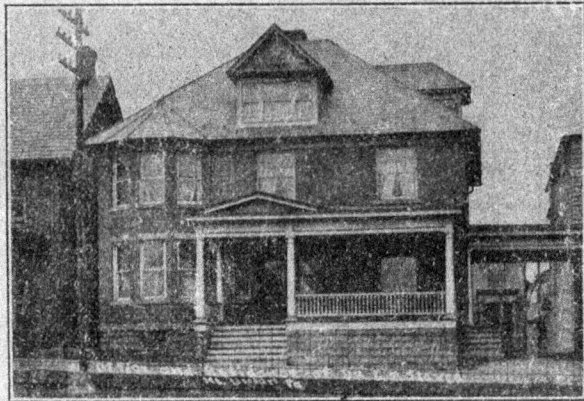

DR. J. C. STEVER, Mount Union, Pa.

The 1911 *Huntingdon Directory*, published the year the hospital opened, lists 14 doctors located in Huntingdon and 14 more dotted about the county. The list is not all-inclusive; only those who paid were included in the classified section. This informative advertisement appeared on the directory's back cover. Dr. Stever's medical expertise extended to "all the ills of the human body," as was common among general practitioners of the era. In the 1890s, Dr. Stever practiced at Three Springs, where he operated a sanitarium that promoted the healing properties of the mineral springs there. (Courtesy of Nancy Shedd.)

Brought to Huntingdon as a physician at the Pennsylvania Industrial Reformatory, Dr. Howard C. Frontz resigned and opened a private practice in 1908. He took a leading role in the instruction of student nurses, teaching the anatomy of all the bodily systems and the handling of infectious diseases. He was one of two Huntingdon doctors elected president of the Pennsylvania Medical Society in the 20th century. (Courtesy of BC.)

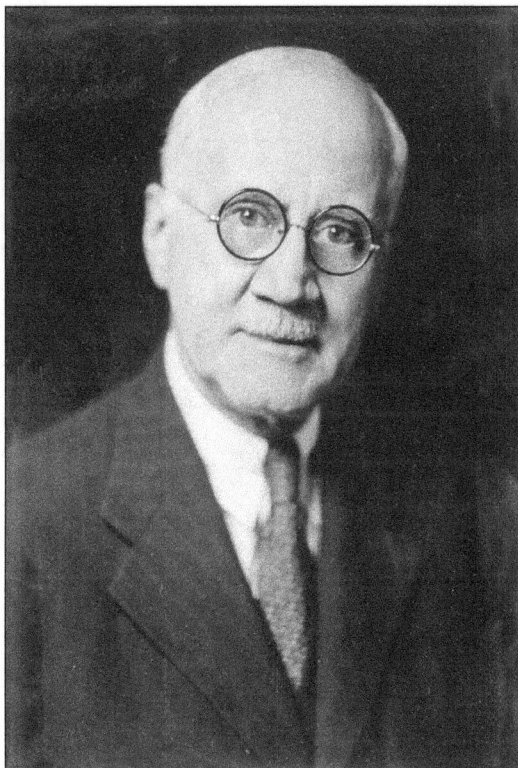

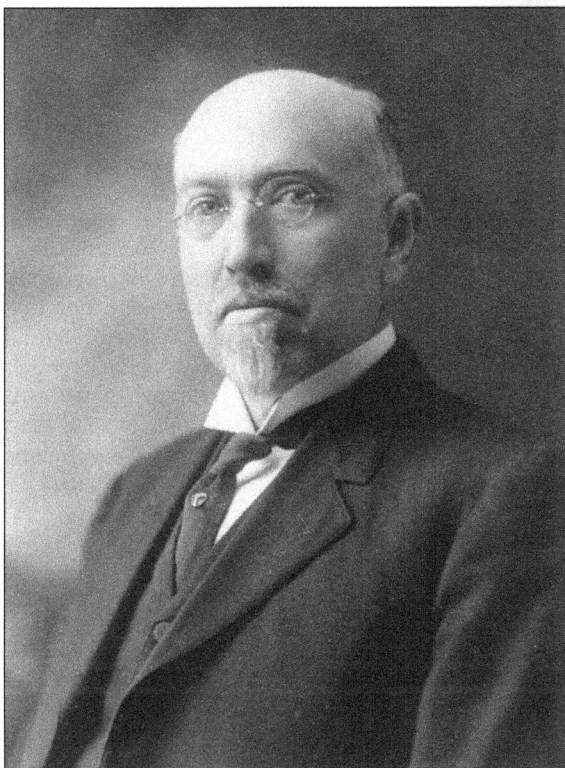

Dr. Henry Clay Chisolm was a student at Vanderbilt University in 1877 when his father, sister, and brother were murdered by the Ku Klux Klan in his native Mississippi, where his father was a judge. After graduating from Hahnemann Medical School in 1888, Chisolm practiced in Huntingdon, where his brother William Wallace Chisolm practiced law. Chiefly a surgeon, Chisolm taught nursing students operating procedures, sterile conditions, and care of sutures and wounds.

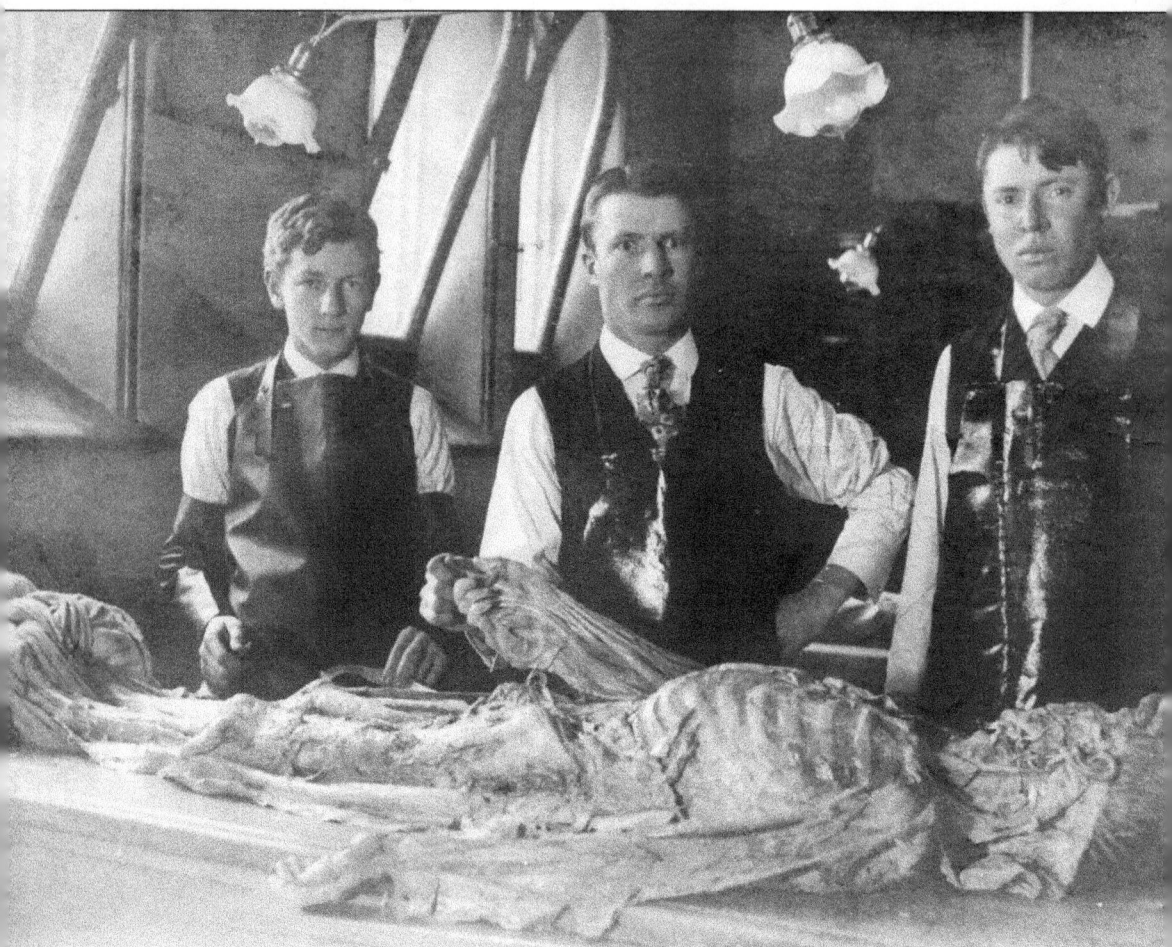

Two of the aspiring doctors seen in this captivating image completed their medical education in 1911. Admission to Hahnemann Medical College, where the photograph was taken, required only high school graduation or "its equivalent" when they matriculated in 1907. Not until 1913 was one year of college required for admission to Philadelphia's many medical schools. A century later, the careful dissection of cadavers may be the only part of a medical student's education that has not changed radically. The same year J. C. Blair Memorial Hospital opened, the influential Flexner Report was published, calling for additional requirements for admission to medical schools and greater emphasis on scientific and hospital-based education, to ensure that medical students had adequate exposure to patients and experience in diagnosing their conditions. Most of Blair Hospital's earliest doctors had already received the quality of education Flexner advocated, having been trained in the respected teaching hospitals of Philadelphia. (Courtesy of Nancy Shedd.)

Until at least the middle of the 20th century, every medical practitioner maintained his own dispensary from which he supplied the medicines required by his patients. Dr. C. A. R. McClain's dispensary was typical: a narrow utilitarian room stocked with bottles of pills and liquids. An 1898 graduate of Medico-Chirurgical College, Dr. McClain served the people of Mount Union for 58 years. (Courtesy of Fred McClain.)

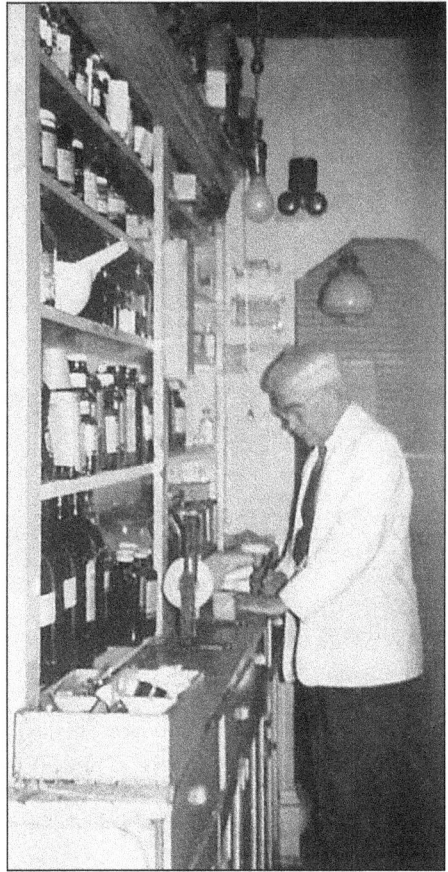

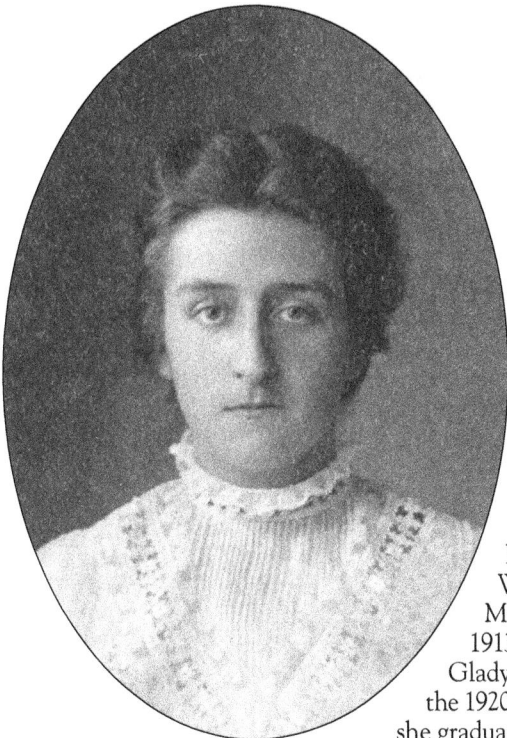

Raised on a Trough Creek Valley farm, Gladys Wright followed her older sister, Nell, to Women's Medical College in Philadelphia, graduating in 1913. Married to dentist Freeman Newlin in 1911, Gladys and her husband practiced in Huntingdon in the 1920s and 1930s. The photograph is from 1907, when she graduated from Huntingdon High School.

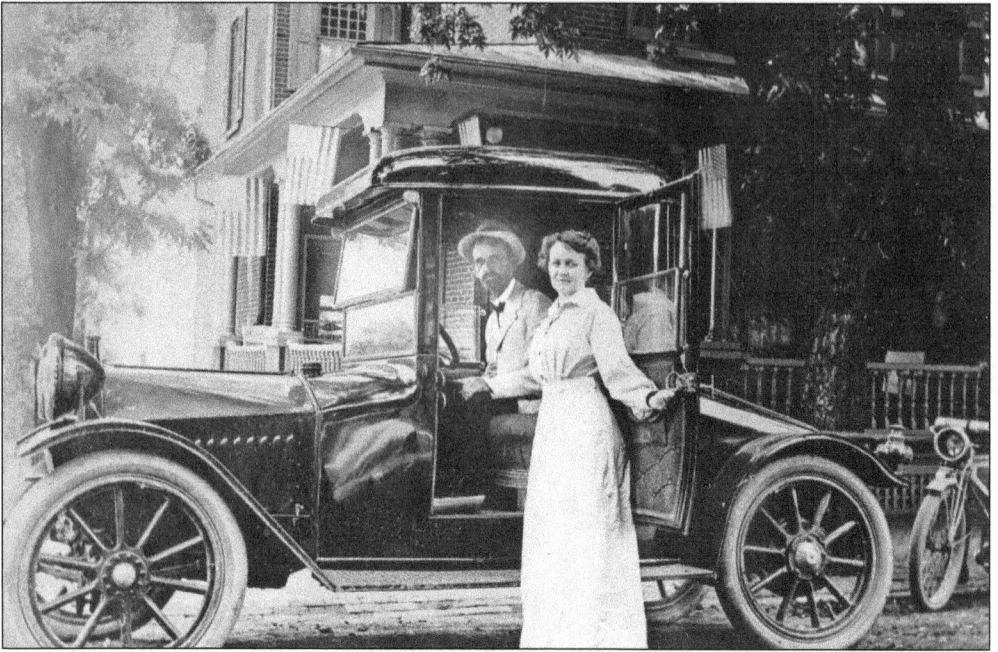

Making house calls was standard practice for doctors through the first half of the 20th century, and doctors were often among the first to exchange their horse and buggy for an automobile to facilitate visiting patients' homes. This image captures Dr. Charles Campbell of Petersburg bidding his wife goodbye as he sets off to call on patients. (Courtesy of Hartslog Museum.)

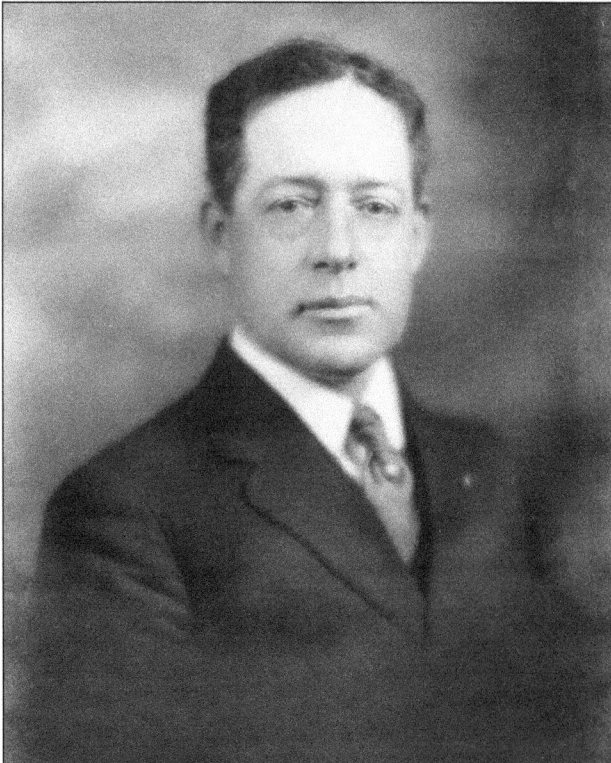

In Alexandria physician Dr. John M. Beck's 40-year career, he claimed to have worn out five fine horses, three Buicks, and two Fords. Some of those miles were logged traveling the county as medical inspector of schools for 25 years. As a general practitioner, Dr. Beck delivered three generations in some families and two sets of triplets. (Courtesy of BC.)

Philadelphia native Dr. John S. Herkness graduated from Hahnemann Medical School in 1910 and became associated with Dr. Chisolm in Huntingdon. Very shortly, however, he moved to Mount Union, where he practiced for 44 years and was deeply involved in community organizations. He was a founder of the Huntingdon County Society for Crippled Children and Adults, now PRIDE.

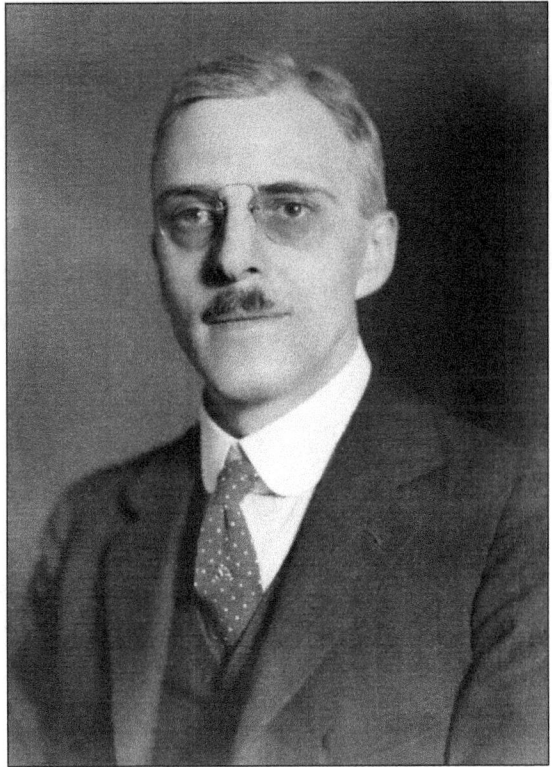

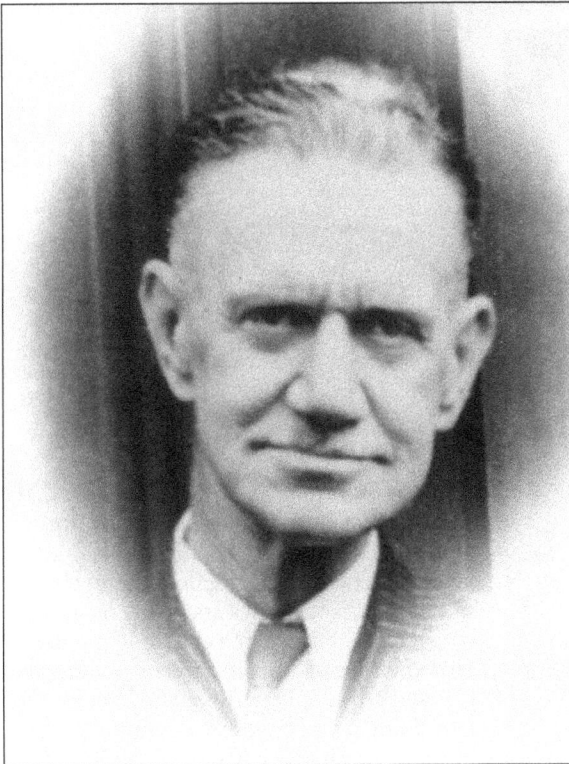

Dr. Harold G. Horton graduated from Philadelphia's Medico-Chirurgical College in 1910 and practiced in Three Springs and Saltillo. Like the doctors on the facing page, Dr. Horton joined Blair Hospital's consulting staff during its first few years. He was active in the Huntingdon County Medical Society, serving a term as president. (Courtesy of BC.)

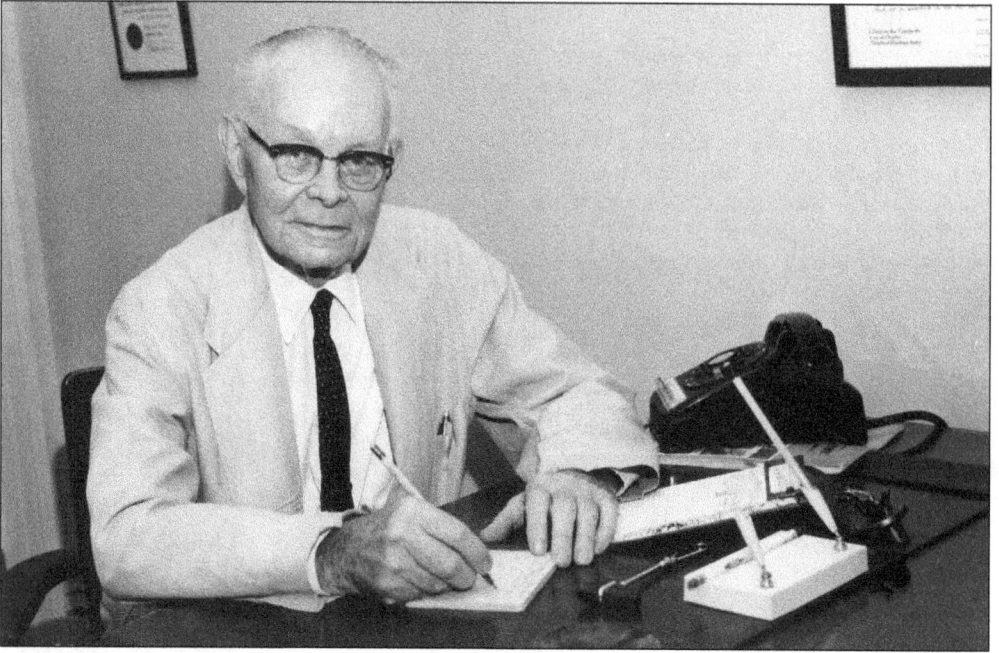

Despite a fine education at Mercersburg, Princeton, and Columbia Medical School, Dr. Fred L. Hutchison was unable to specialize in surgery when he began to practice in Huntingdon. Even with two postgraduate years of training in surgery, he began as a general practitioner. This photograph accompanied a 1966 article in *The Daily News* marking Hutchison's 50 years in practice, all of them at J. C. Blair. (Courtesy of BC.)

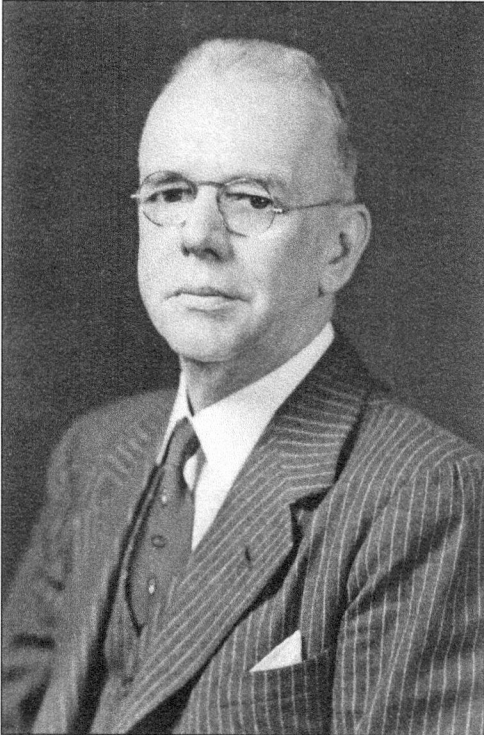

Dr. Cloy G. Brumbaugh was a Juniata College graduate with a year of study in biology at the University of Pennsylvania before entering medical school there. He specialized in obstetrics and gynecology, in which he also instructed the student nurses. His office at 805 Mifflin Street was occupied previously by Dr. Fetterhoof and later by Drs. Fillman and Savory—a century of care in the same quarters. (Courtesy of BC.)

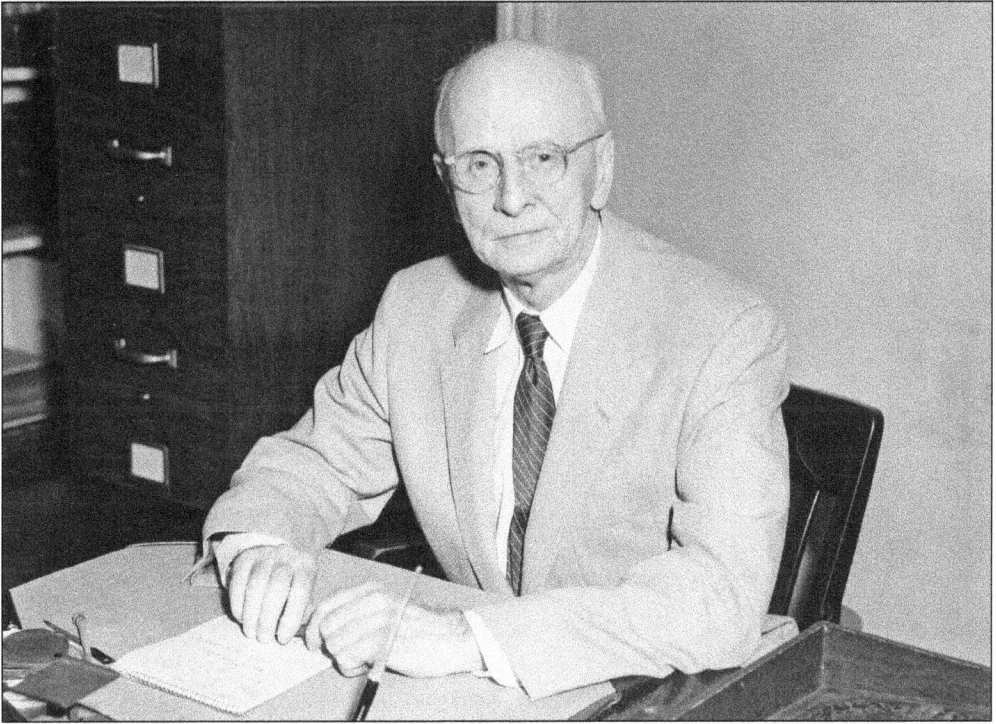

After studies at Penn State and in his father's law office, John M. Keichline graduated from American Medical Missionary College and practiced for three years in Egypt. Returning home, he settled in Petersburg and was on Blair Hospital's consulting staff for x-ray, pathology, and anesthesia. Graduate study in x-ray, following World War I service, qualified him to head the hospital's radiology department and to join the premier radiology societies. (Courtesy of BC.)

Barter was a time-honored method of payment of all kinds of debts, although Mr. Belknap considered the arrangement a courtesy to him. Dr. Keichline probably considered it mutually beneficial; fresh eggs were delivered to his door every week for four months. The agreement may have been unusual in the doctor's experience, as he took care to preserve this record of it.

Dr. J. M. Keichline,
Huntingdon, Penna.

Dear Doctor:–

As payment of your bill, I have delivered eggs as follows.

June	25	2	Dozen @ 23¢	.46
July	2	1	" " 23	.23
"	10	2	" " 24	.48
"	17	1	" " 24	.24
"	24	2	" " 30	.60
Aug.	7	2	" " 32	.64
"	14	1	" " 32	.32
"	21	2	" " 33	.66
"	28	1	" " 33	.33
Sept.	4	2	" " 33	.66
"	11	2	" " 33	.66
"	18	2	" " 33	.66
"	25	2	" " 33	.66
Oct.	2	2	" " 35	.70
"	9	2	" " 35	.70
"	16	2	" " 37.5	.75
"	23	2	" " 40	.80
"	30	1	" " 40	.40
	Cash			.05

$10.00

I wish to thank you very much for the work you have done, the courtesy of waiting for your pay, and for the priviledge you have extended to me of paying as I have.

Sincerely,

R. K. Belknap

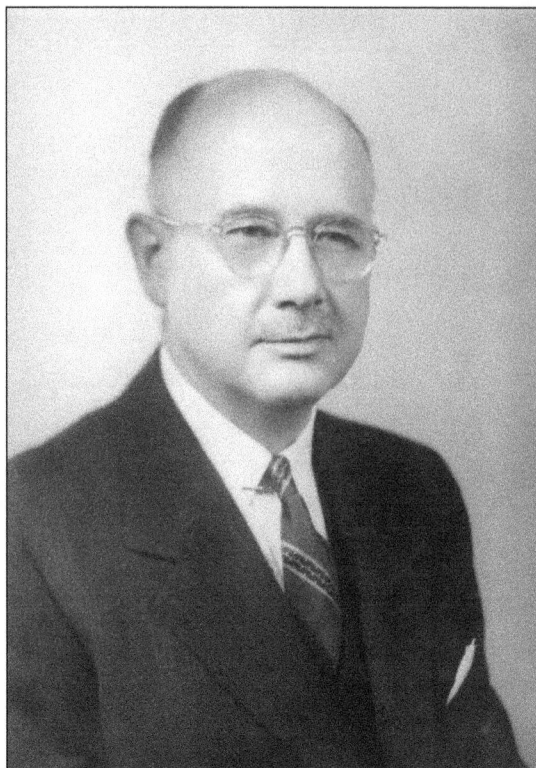

While engaged in a regular medical practice, Dr. Charles R. Reiners filled the post of hospital pathologist. He was a 1913 graduate of the University of Pennsylvania Medical School. Stories survive about the sheep Dr. Reiners kept at the hospital. It is likely he used sheep blood to culture streptococcus and staphylococcus bacteria in the laboratory. He berated the nurses for overfeeding the sheep, which they considered pets. (Courtesy of BC.)

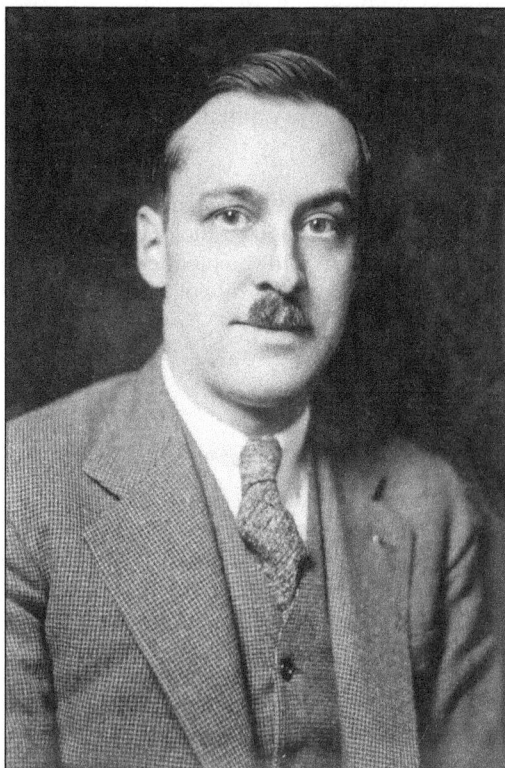

Dr. William A. Doebele came to Huntingdon around 1920, following graduation from medical school and service in the U.S. Navy. He served at the Philadelphia Naval Yard during the 1918 influenza epidemic, which killed 50 million people worldwide, far surpassing the 13 million estimated casualties of World War I. Dr. Doebele hoped to practice surgery in Huntingdon, but, like others, had to engage in general practice. (Courtesy of BC.)

A longtime Mount Union physician was Dr. William J. Campbell, a Shirley Township native who taught school to earn money for further education. He eventually enrolled at Medico-Chirurgical College in Philadelphia, graduating in 1893. Though an early automobile owner, Campbell loved to tell of practicing medicine in the horse-and-buggy days. He was an organizer and lifelong director of First National Bank of Mount Union. (Courtesy of BC.)

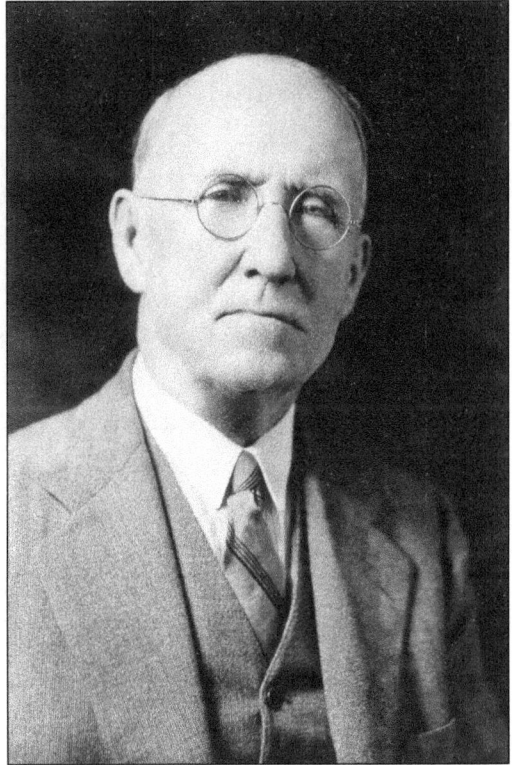

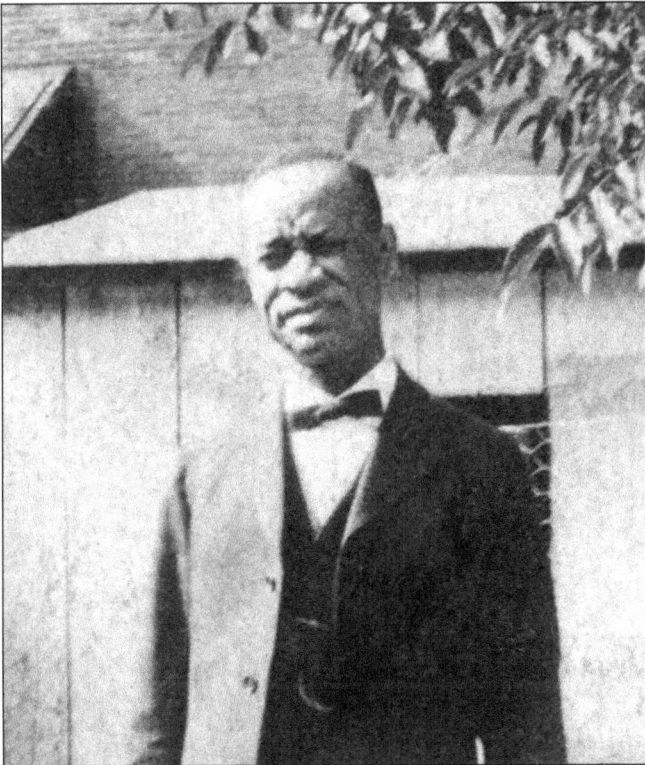

Dr. Charles S. Brooks was a 1910 graduate of Howard University's School of Medicine. He came to Mount Union in 1936, became active in the community, and enjoyed a wide circle of friends and patients. He was once able to calm the fears of a mother whose young son was having trouble walking. Did he have polio? No, Dr. Brooks assured her, he's just drunk. (Courtesy of BC.)

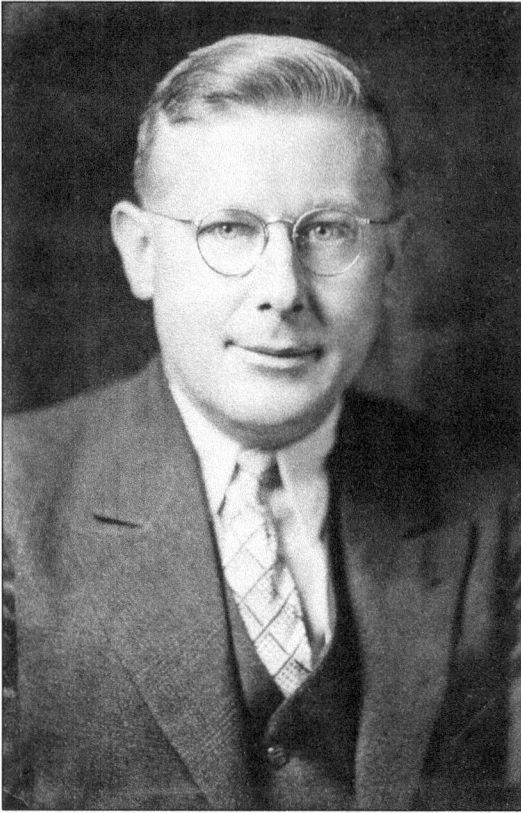

A graduate of Temple University Medical School, Dr. Walter Orthner came to Huntingdon in 1931. At the height of the baby boom following World War II, Dr. Orthner's practice was also booming. One memorable day, he delivered six babies to four mothers in 79 minutes. The date was July 21, 1947; the six babies included the first set of triplets born at J. C. Blair Memorial Hospital. The triplets' birth was front-page news; *The Daily News* called Orthner "Huntingdon County's Dr. Dafoe," referring to the Canadian doctor who delivered the Dionne quintuplets in 1934. The triplets were children of Mr. and Mrs. William Faulkner of Mount Union. Unfortunately, little Joan lived only a day. Pictured are the surviving twins—Jean Faulkner of Aurora, Colorado, and Joe Faulkner, now of Pittsburgh. (Left, courtesy of BC; below, courtesy of Jean Faulkner.)

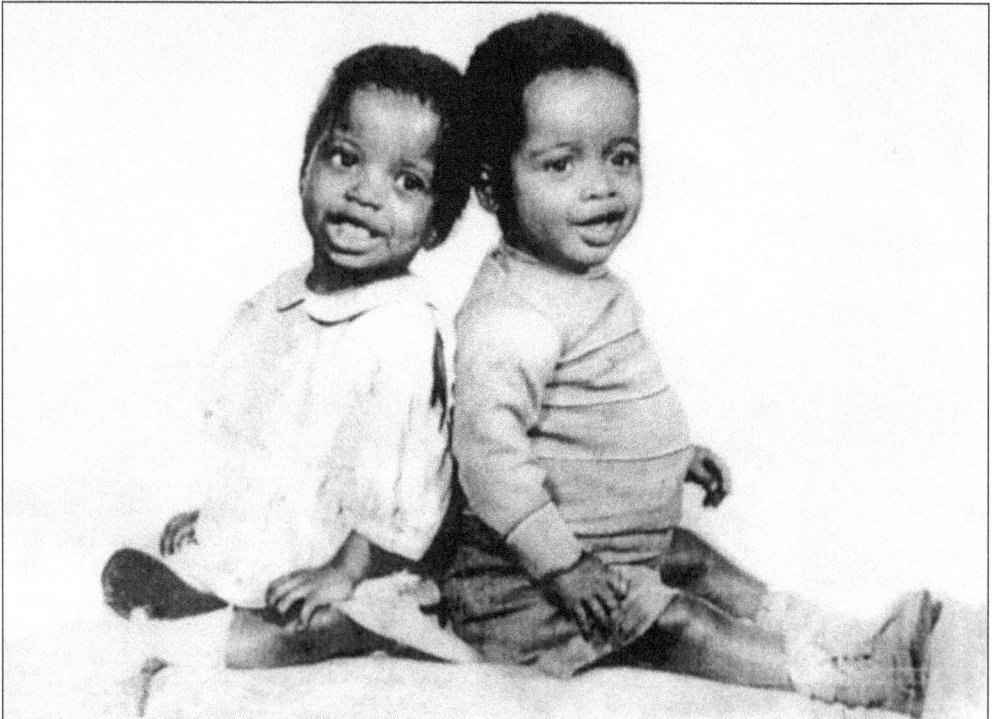

Dr. William B. West, a graduate of Huntingdon High School, Juniata College, and Jefferson Medical School, opened his Huntingdon office in 1934. He was one of six doctors who joined the hospital staff in the 1930s, replacing older staff. Dr. West was an officer in many community and medical organizations; he served on the Huntingdon School Board for 25 years and was elected president of the Pennsylvania Medical Society. (Courtesy of TDN.)

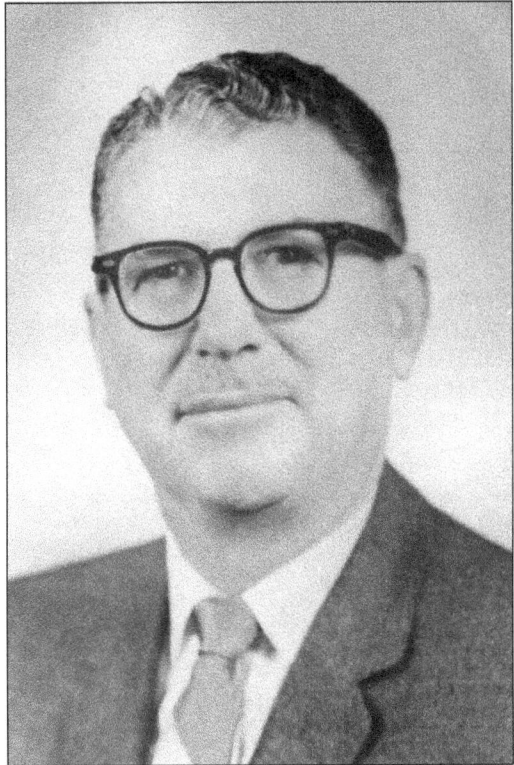

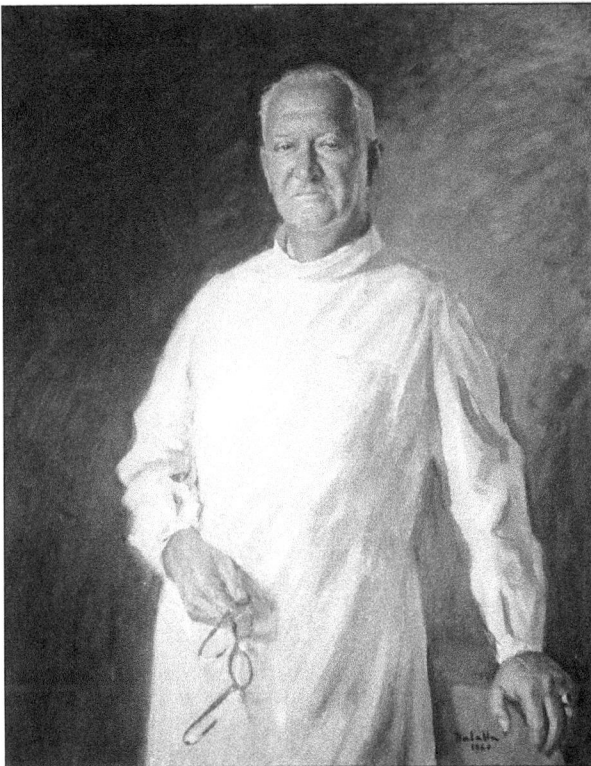

Also a Huntingdon native, Dr. Frederic H. Steele attended the same schools as Dr. West and joined Dr. Fred Hutchison in the practice of surgery in 1936. He entered military service in 1941, heading surgical units in hospitals in Virginia and in England before his discharge in 1945. This striking portrait was painted around 1960 and was given by his family to the hospital. (Photograph by Linda Cutshall.)

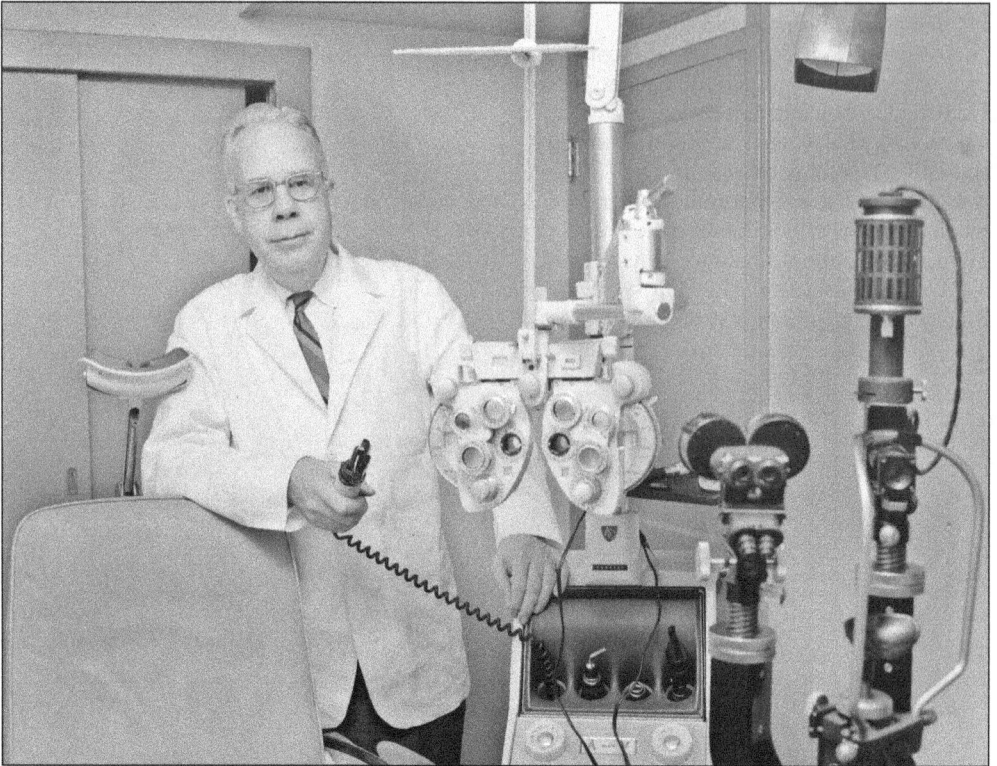

A 1936 graduate of the University of Pittsburgh Medical School, Dr. H. Ford Clark took postgraduate studies in ophthalmology and otolaryngology and opened his Huntingdon practice in 1937. Active in his church and community, he volunteered for three tours of duty on the USS *Hope*, a medical ship serving poor nations. In 1969, Dr. Clark became president of the Pennsylvania Academy of Ophthalmology and Otolaryngology.

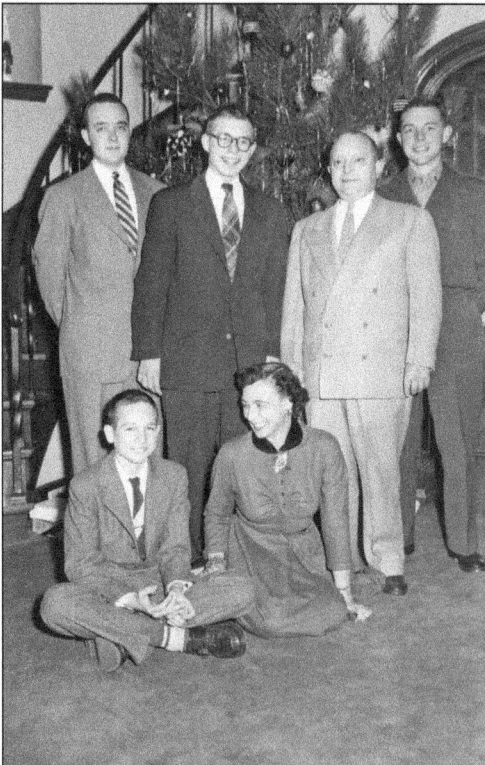

In 1935, almost 10 years after graduation from Jefferson Medical School, Dr. Francis S. Mainzer joined the staff of J.C. Blair Memorial Hospital as an experienced surgeon. His 25-year career there included three-and-half years of military service during World War II. The Mainzer family photograph was a 1950s Christmas card. Dr. Mainzer's two oldest sons followed him into medicine. (Courtesy of the Schucker Estate.)

Following his 1937 graduation from Hahnemann Medical College, Dr. William B. Patterson undertook residencies in pathology and in cardiology with noted cardiologist Dr. Paul Dudley White. White particularly advocated use of the electrocardiogram in diagnosing heart ailments. In 1961, Dr. Patterson and Mrs. Betty Migatulski inspected a new $895 electrocardiograph machine, purchased for the hospital by the Huntingdon County Heart Association.

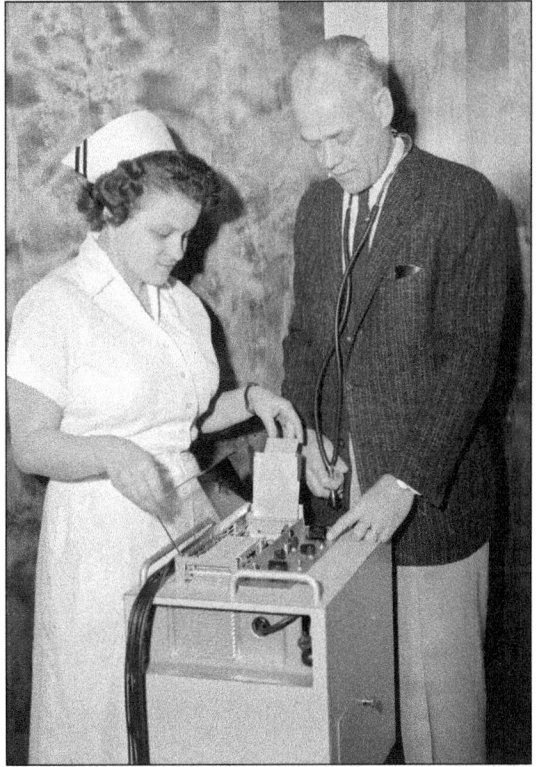

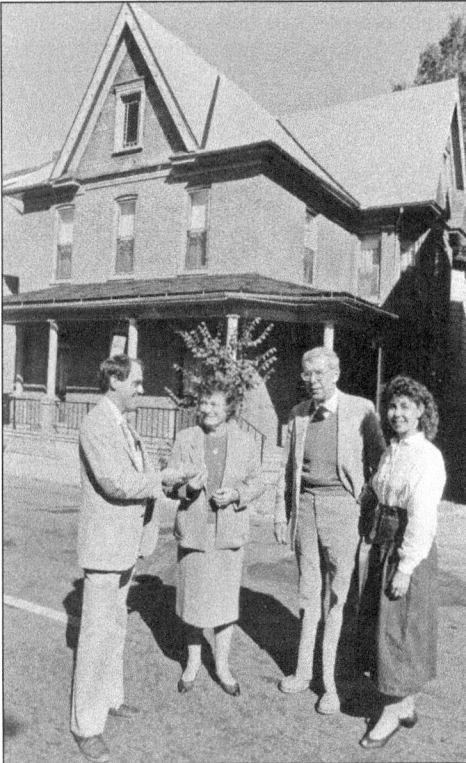

As an internist, trained at Temple University School of Medicine and the Cleveland Clinic, Dr. Robert H. Beck shared Dr. Patterson's interest in treating heart patients. His office was at 923 Mifflin Street, seen here behind Dr. and Mrs. Beck, from 1946 until his retirement in 1984. His interest in local history led Dr. Beck to collect many of the photographs used in this chapter.

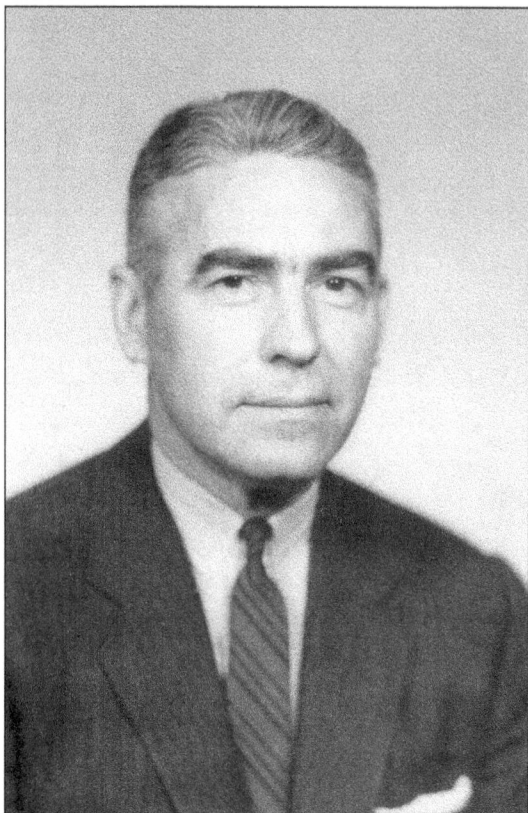

A native of Pittsburgh and a 1936 graduate of the University of Pittsburgh Medical School, Dr. John B. Fillman had five years of advanced study in obstetrics and gynecology in Pittsburgh before coming to Huntingdon in 1941. He took over the practice and office of Dr. Cloy Brumbaugh, who died that year at age 57. (Courtesy of TDN.)

Following graduation from Jefferson Medical College in 1941, Dr. Charles L. Schucker served in the U.S. Army for four years. In 1948, he purchased the medical practice of Dr. William A. Doebele, with whom he had been associated. After further study at his alma mater, Dr. Schucker specialized in obstetrics and gynecology. (Courtesy of the Schucker Estate.)

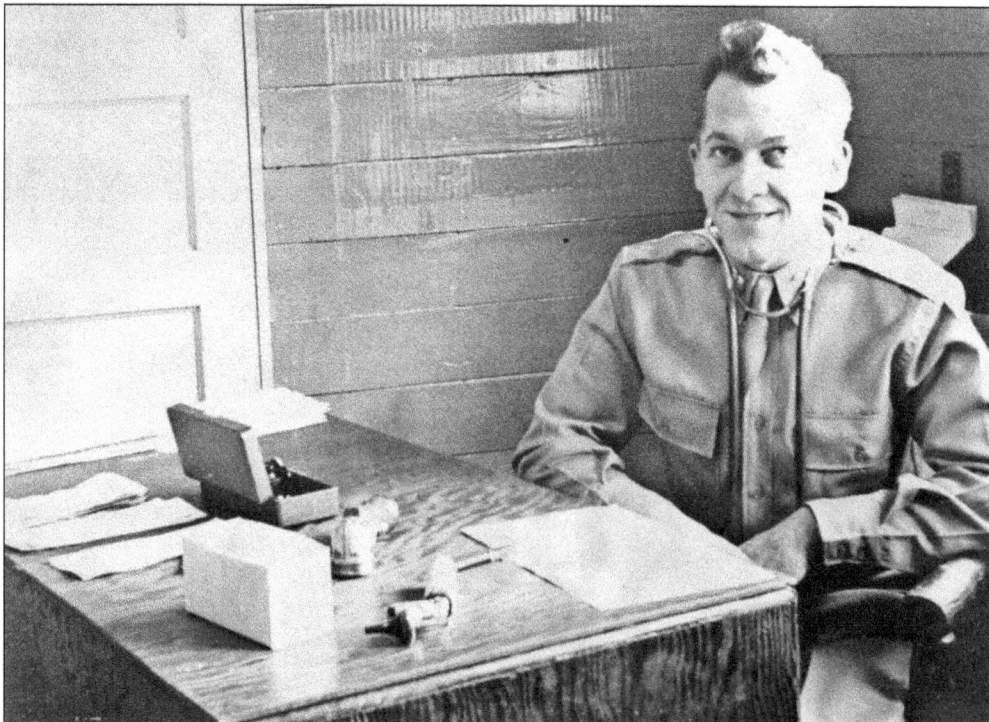

A 1941 Huntingdon High School graduate, Dr. William W. Schock enlisted in the V-12 program, which allowed prospective doctors to complete their education before being drafted into military service. Thus, he was not called to serve until the Korean Conflict, when he had to leave his newly established pediatrics practice for two years. Dr. Schock's was the first local practice to focus entirely on children. (Courtesy of TDN.)

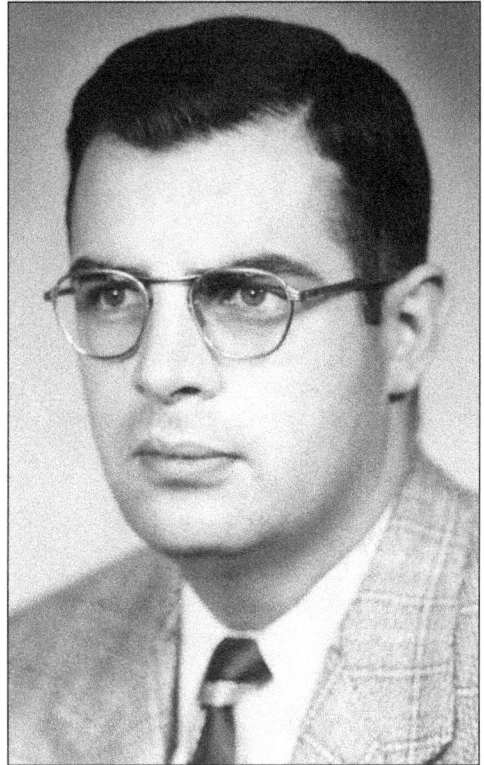

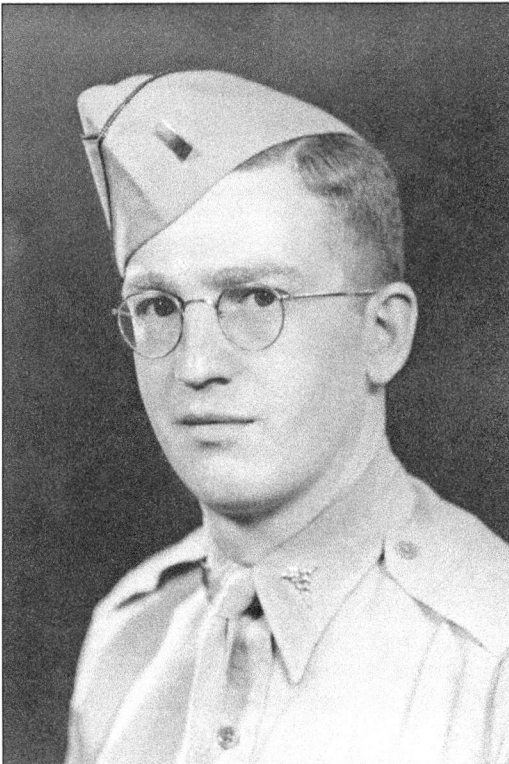

Dr. Fred H. McClain Jr. joined his grandfather, Dr. C. A. R. McClain, in the practice of medicine in 1947, following discharge from military service. A 1944 graduate of the University of Pennsylvania School of Medicine, Dr. McClain became the clinician and medical director of the Mount Union Area Medical Center from 1979, when it opened, to his retirement in 1988. (Courtesy of Fred McClain.)

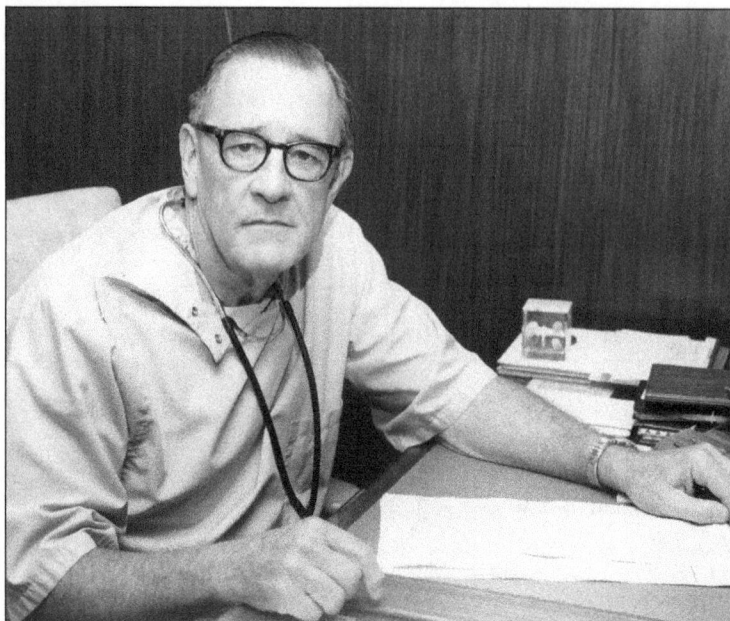

Dr. Harry H. Negley began to practice medicine in Alexandria in 1935 and, in 1947, moved his practice to Huntingdon. A 1934 graduate of the University of Pittsburgh School of Medicine, Dr. Negley was elected Huntingdon County coroner in 1965, serving until his death in 1980. (Courtesy of Hartslog Museum.)

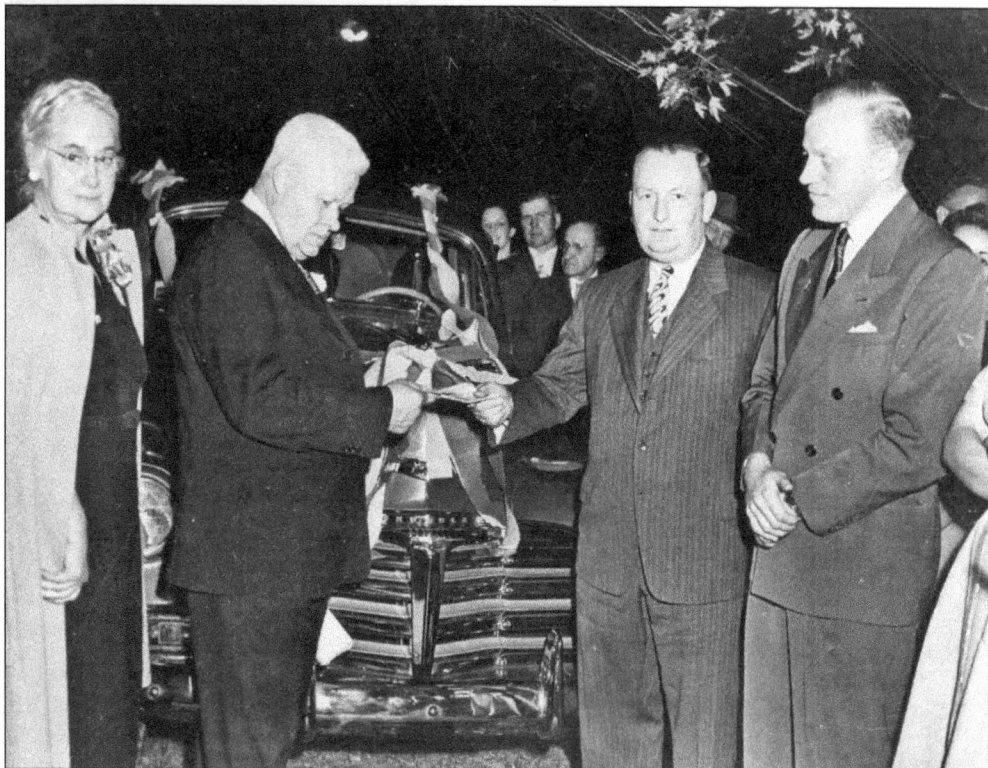

In 1948, around 300 Warriors Mark neighbors of Dr. Harry C. Wilson paid tribute to the doctor who had served them for 40 years, since graduating from Baltimore College of Physicians and Surgeons in 1908. Following speeches of appreciation by community representatives and fellow doctors, Dr. Wilson was presented with a new Chevrolet sedan. Pictured are, from left to right, Mrs. and Dr. Wilson, Robert Harpster, and Rev. Paul Myers. (Courtesy of BC.)

A 1947 graduate of the University of Pennsylvania Medical School, with specialized training in surgery, Dr. Charles Robert Reiners Jr. was assigned to a MASH unit during the Korean Conflict. He completed his residency after military service, returning to Huntingdon in 1960. The photograph shows Reiners as toastmaster at a retirement dinner in 1977 for 3-11 shift supervisor Marie Daschbach (front); Julia Craig looks on. (Courtesy of TDN.)

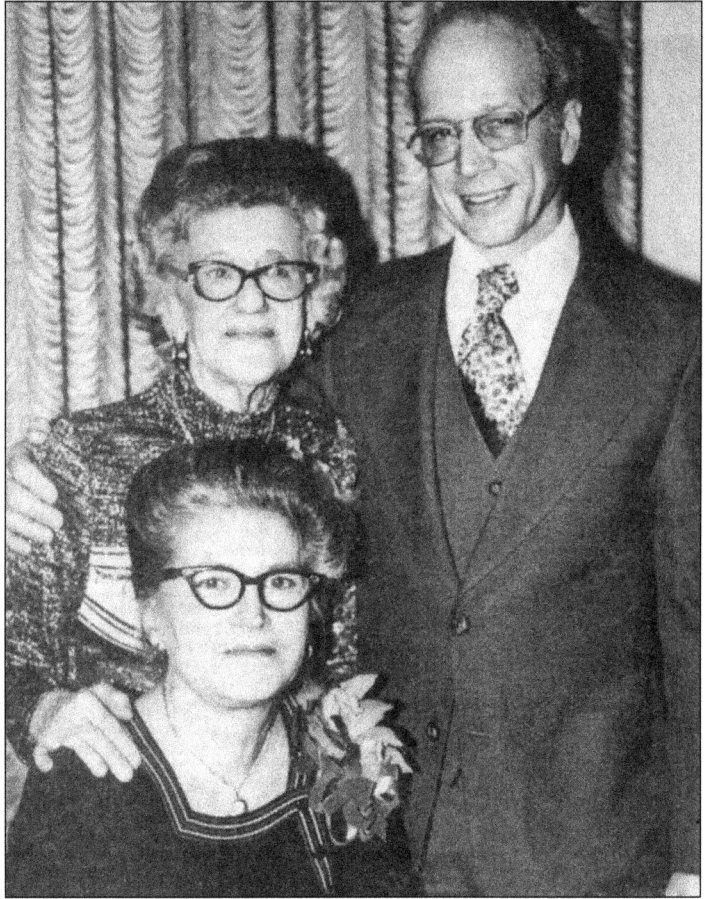

While attached to a MASH unit in Korea, Dr. Burgess A. Smith was awarded the Distinguished Flying Cross, Bronze Stars, and Meritorious Service Medal for his part in air rescue missions behind enemy lines. Earlier he served two years as a medical corpsman in World War II. In this 1959 photograph, the year Smith came to Huntingdon, he explains to hospital administrator Richard Cummings how a defibrillator works.

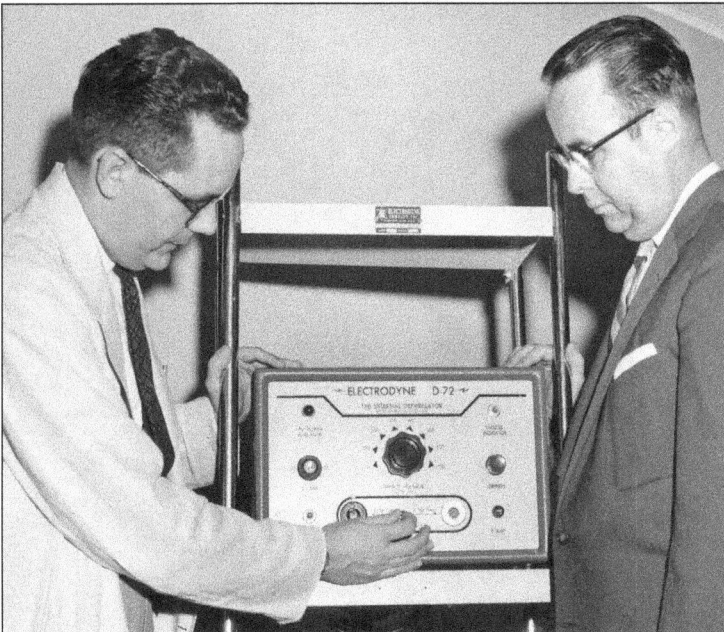

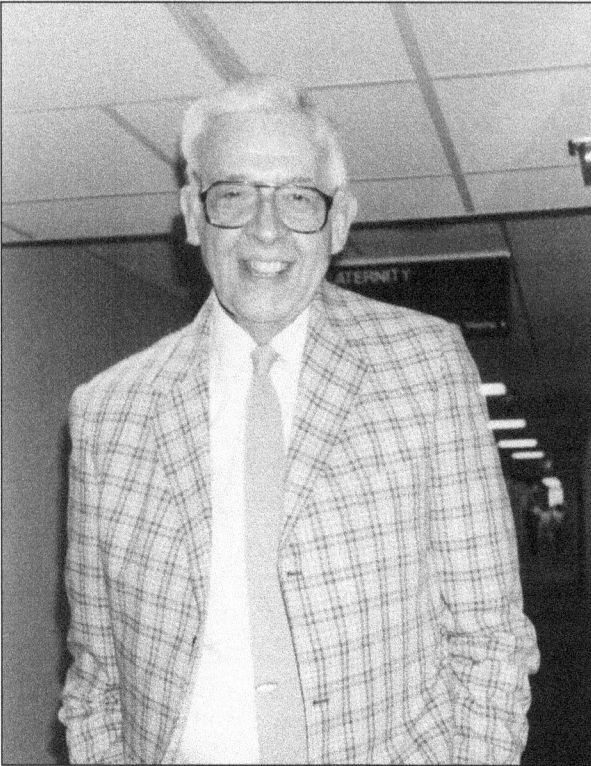

In 1953, Dr. Philip S. Dunn opened his practice in the Sixth Street office vacated by Dr. Schucker, who was returning to school for specialized training. Dr. Dunn saw combat in Europe during World War II before returning to college and earning his medical degree at Jefferson Medical College in 1952. This "true gentleman," as so many characterize him, served patients and community for almost 40 years, retiring in 1991. (Courtesy of Dr. Philip S. Dunn.)

Saltillo native Dr. Walter B. Watkin Sr. graduated from Juniata College and Jefferson Medical School before opening an office in his hometown in 1940. "Dr. Sonny," as he was fondly called, was physician to residents of the Shirley Home for the Aged from 1969 to 1980 and served as an emergency department physician from 1969 to 1984. (Courtesy of BC.)

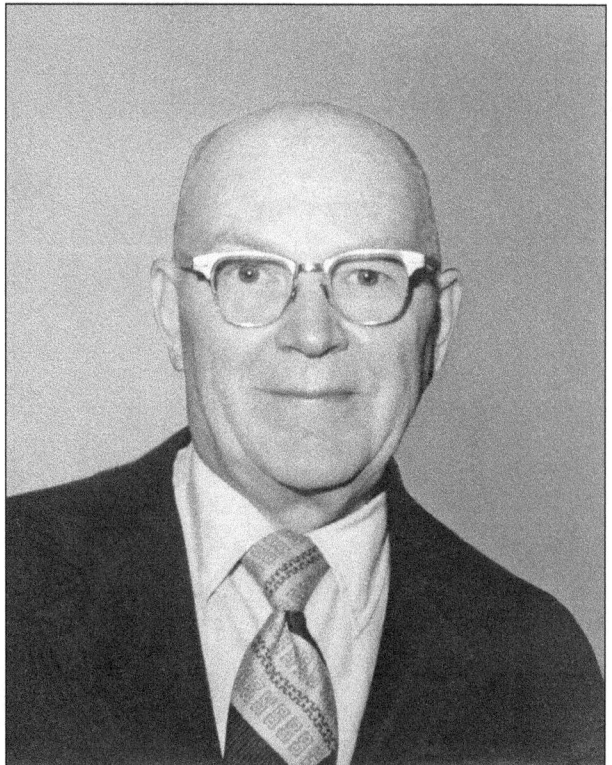

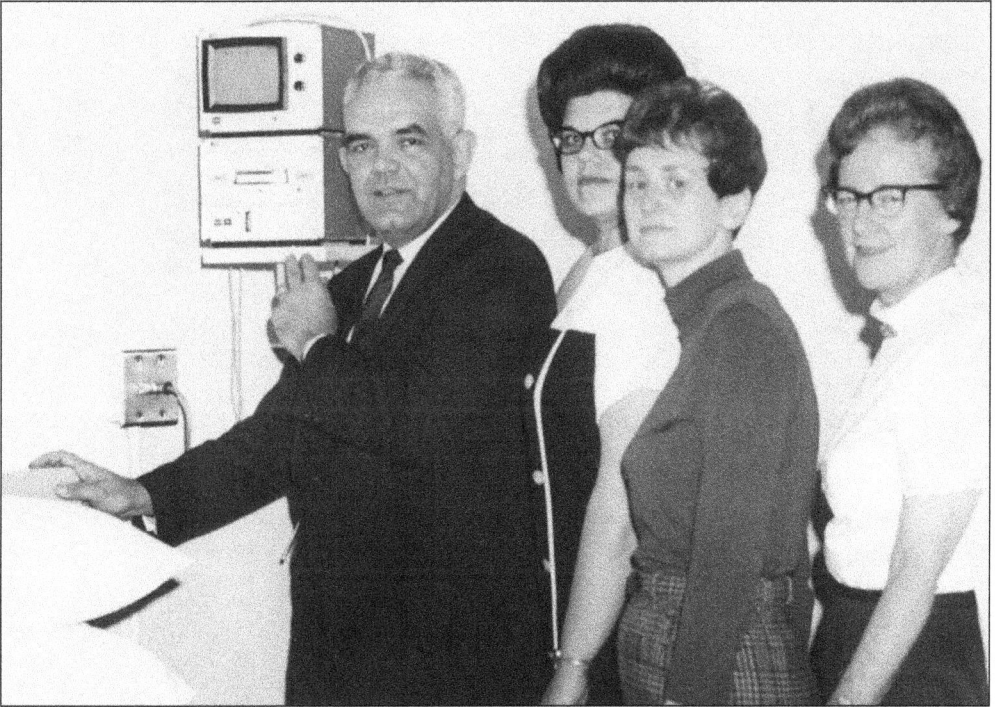

Dr. Theodore D. Whitsel represented the hospital's Special Care Unit committee at the opening of the first intensive care unit in May 1969. (Others pictured represented agencies that funded the unit.) A graduate of the University of Pennsylvania Medical School in 1949, Dr. Whitsel was certified in internal medicine in 1958. He practiced in Huntingdon from 1960 until his retirement in 1988.

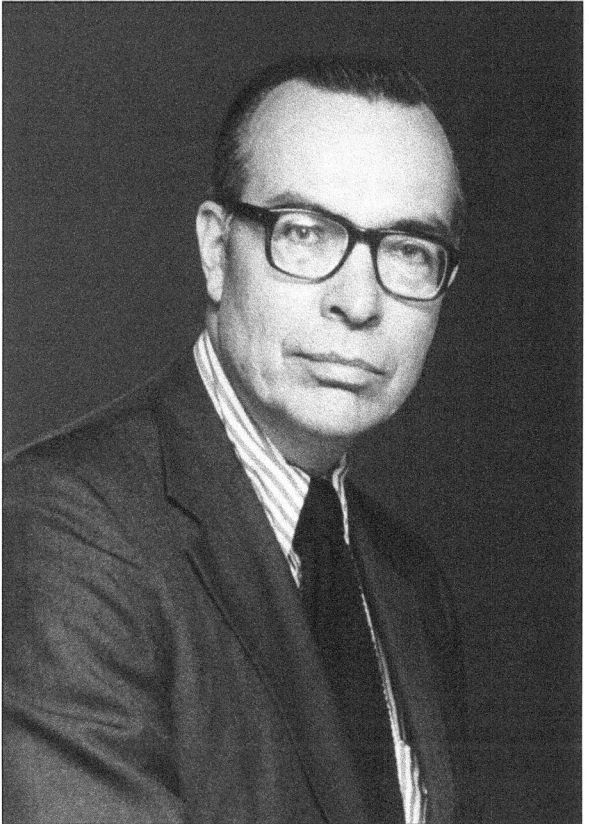

Dr. Frederick E. Wawrose was added to the hospital staff in 1970 to head the new Department of Psychiatry. A 1954 graduate of the University of Pennsylvania Medical School, he was board certified in both adult and child psychiatry. The department he launched, now known as Behavioral Health Services, treats nearly 400 children and adults, both inpatients and outpatients, and conducts more than 600 assessments annually.

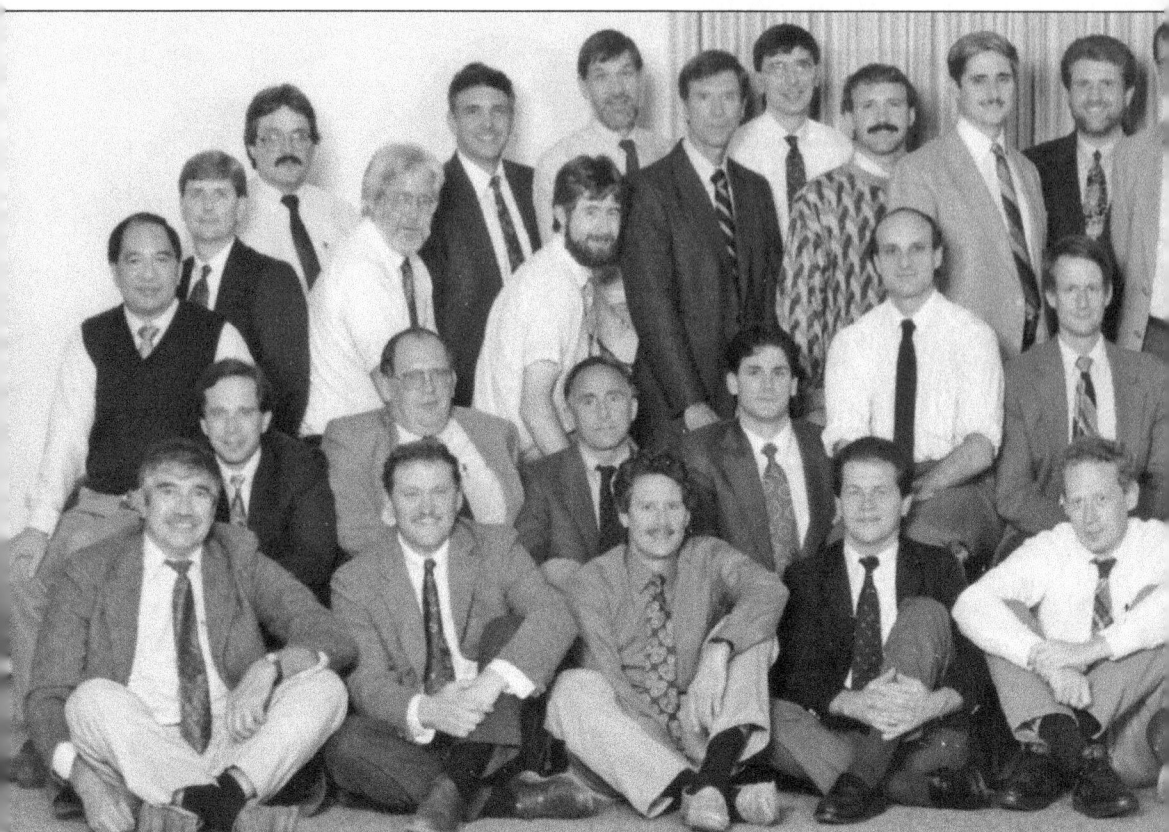

Forty-four doctors on the medical staff of J. C. Blair Memorial Hospital assembled in 1993 for this group photograph. From left to right are (first row) David Jacobson, Brian Hoover, Gary Wertman, Allen Strunk, James Schall, Richard DiDonato, Kenneth Lee, Robert Lamey, William Bressler, and David Miller; (second row, beginning with man in sleeveless sweater) Antonio Colmenar, Michael Gaugler, John Maylock, David Zeigler, Michael Cesare, John D'Andrea, Theodore Shively, Julann Bower (medical secretary), George Thorpe, James Savory, Scott Grugan, Philip

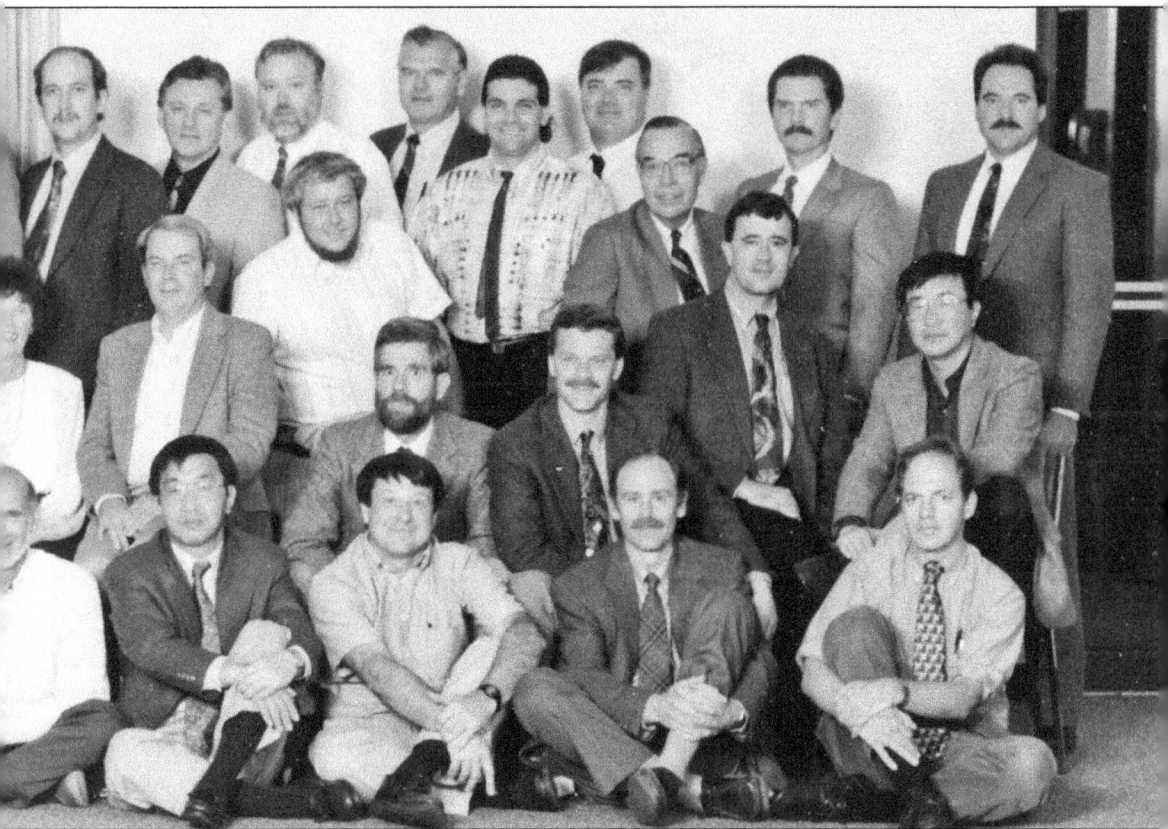

Shoaf, and Kevin Lee. Visible in the back are Keith Waddle, Mark Minor, Richard Buza, Ronald Costa, William Depp-Hutchison, David Clymer, Richard Ewell, James Sioma, Daniel Delp, Christopher Patitsas, Ronald Long, Allen Ettenger, Keith Sutton, Nick Poltawec, Bruce Lidston, James Hayden, Winfried Berger, Brett Acker, Frederick Jones, Frederick Wawrose, Bradley Pifalo, and James Hardesty.

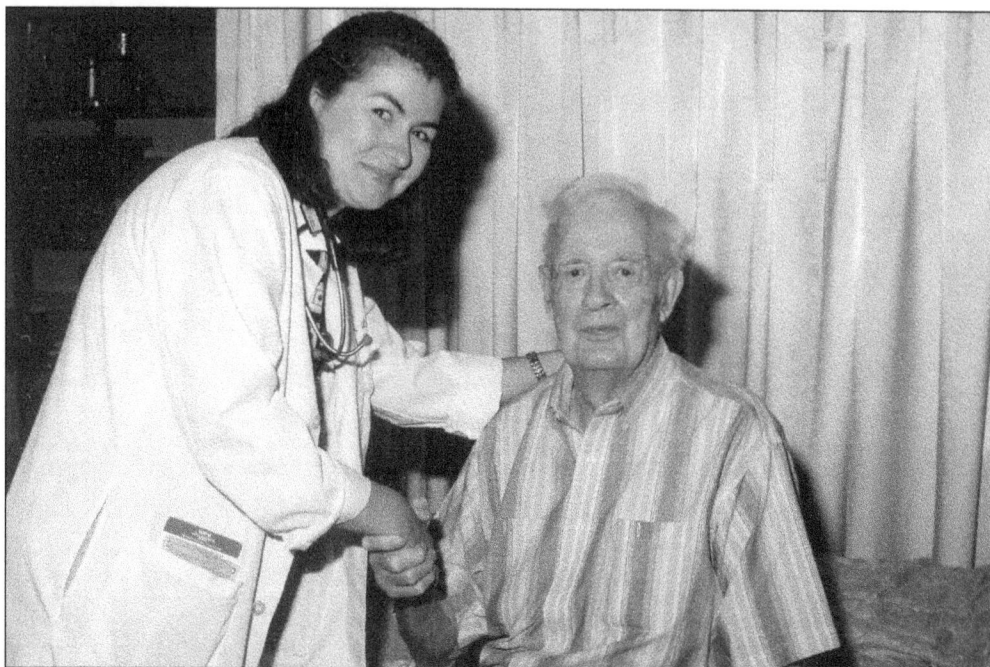

Before Dr. Tracy Lillie saw her first patient at the Juniata Valley Medical Center in Alexandria in 1999, she called on 91-year-old Dr. Donald Malcolm, who was instrumental in seeing the center open its doors in 1972. The medical centers that sprang up around the county in the 1970s were staffed by young physicians and dentists from the National Health Service Corps, which sent doctors to underserved rural areas.

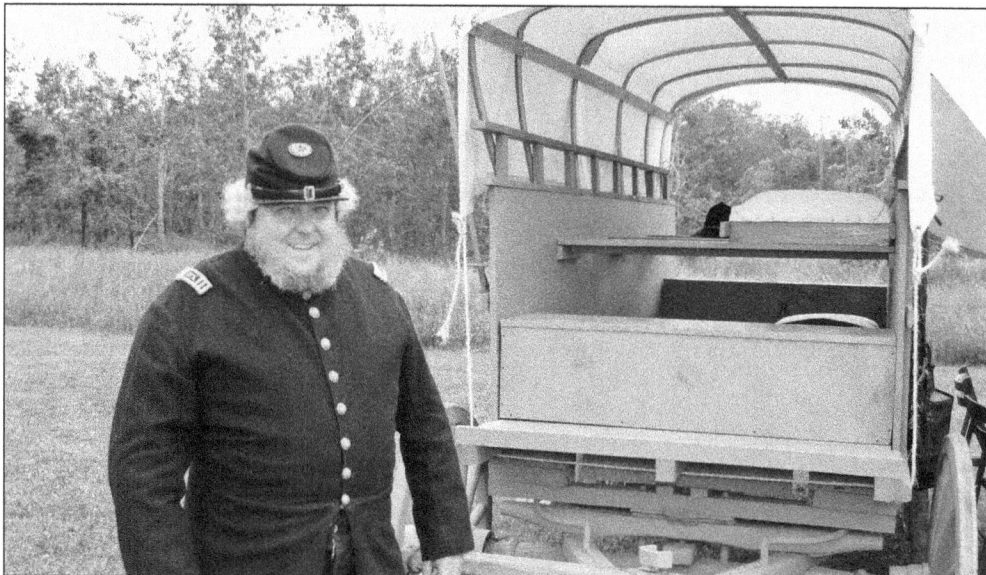

In 2003, Dr. James B. Hayden celebrated the Broad Top Area Medical Center's 30th anniversary in his Civil War reenactor uniform, with his Civil War–era ambulance. Dr. Hayden has been affiliated with the Broad Top center since 1986. He was joined there in 1991 by Dr. Brett L. Acker, now in the emergency department, and in 1997 by Dr. Dominick Kistler, now a hospitalist at Blair. (Courtesy of Adam Watson.)

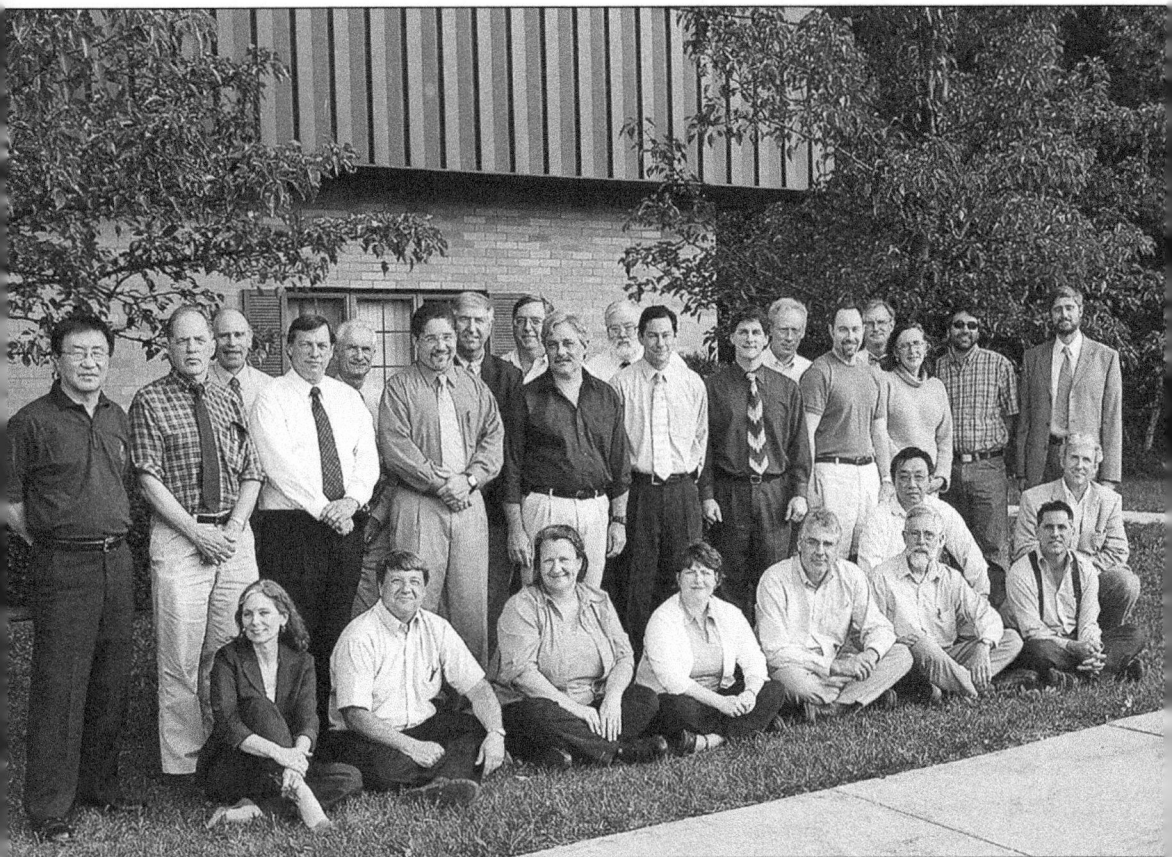

This photograph of Blair Hospital's staff doctors was taken in 2006. Pictured are, from left to right, (seated) Laurie Kile, Robert Lamey, Maria Pettinger, Amy Swindell, Martin Keeney, James Savory, Kenneth Lee, Harry Kamerow, and Daniel Delp; (standing) Kevin Lee, David Miller, William Bressler, Ralph Aldinger, Steven Draskoczy, Frank Hamlett, Bruce Thomas, Francis Pessolano, Mark Minor, Bruce Lidston, Frank Berkey, Michael Cesare, James Schall, James Mansberger, Allen Ettenger, Molly Ettenger, Dominick Kistler, and Christopher Patitsas. A number of doctors who came to the area in the 1970s and 1980s have recently retired or are approaching retirement. The hospital is once again engaged in a generational recruitment campaign. This one involves another generational shift: most young doctors do not want to operate individual practices but expect to join a group such as the newly created J. C. Blair Medical Services. This arm of J. C. Blair Health System provides management services to physicians and has seen recent success in recruiting new doctors.

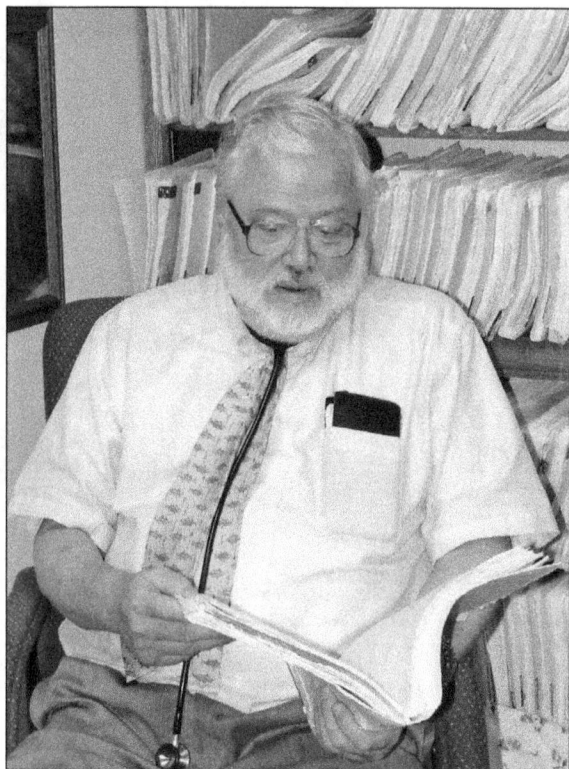

Fall 2009 was tough for patients of longtime Huntingdon physicians Bruce Lidston and Jim Savory. Dr. Lidston retired from his pediatrics practice after 34 years, and Dr. Savory closed his office after 29 years. Trained at Cornell and Cincinnati Children's Hospital, Dr. Lidston served in the U.S. Navy before coming to Huntingdon. Looking back on his career, he remembered advances in children's immunizations and the diagnostic capabilities of ultrasound and CT scanning. (Courtesy of TDN.)

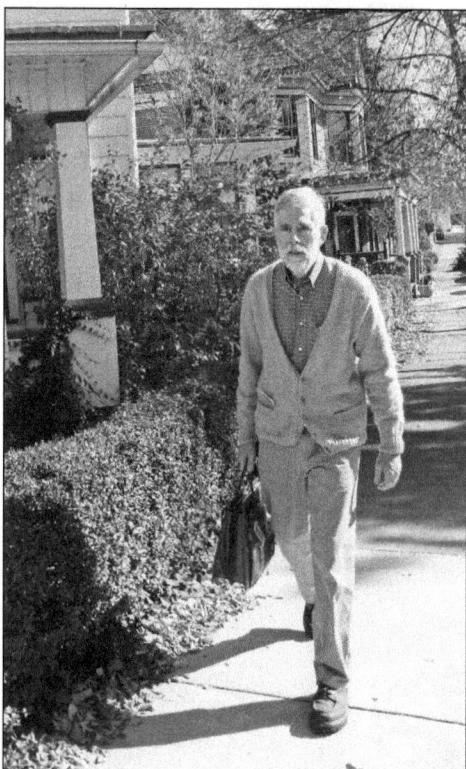

Dr. Savory took his medical training at the University of Michigan and worked for Indian Health Services in Oklahoma before coming to Huntingdon. An internist, Dr. Savory and his wife and receptionist, Judy, presided over an office filled with local history and medical memorabilia, keeping waiting patients relaxed despite a sign that cautioned "Beware of the doc." (Courtesy of TDN.)

Six

BUILDINGS

From 1911 until the ground breaking in 1949 for a major expansion, no additions had been made to J. C. Blair Memorial Hospital's original building. Facilities that provided adequate capacity and technology through the early decades had become crowded and outdated by the late 1940s. A sudden rise in the institution's daily population—caused by a bumper week in the postwar baby boom or by a train wreck near Petersburg—threatened the hospital's ability to meet the medical needs of those it had pledged to serve. The situation was not just inconvenient; it could be dangerous.

Leon Houck, the hospital's first administrator, hired in 1946, focused on the urgent need for a major addition. A campaign to raise more than $1 million, coming on the heels of the Depression and World War II, was a tall order. But Houck and the trustees, led by Judge Thomas F. Bailey, past president, and Chalmers B. Miller, newly elected president, were up to the task. No doubt many donors, or their family members, had occupied beds in the halls when there was no room elsewhere and, therefore, had experienced firsthand how urgent the need was.

The hospital took a huge leap forward with its first large expansion, more than doubling in size, updating technologies, and creating room for future growth. But by the late 1960s, planning was underway to expand the emergency department, to add an acute care wing, and to attach a county-owned nursing care facility to the hospital—all of which were completed in 1972.

Projects in the 1980s and 1990s have brought the hospital to its present configuration, with a campus that includes physicians' offices, education classrooms, physical therapy facilities, and a helipad. Changing practices in medical care and in its modes of delivery challenge Blair Hospital to continually upgrade its facilities to satisfy the needs and expectations of both doctors and patients.

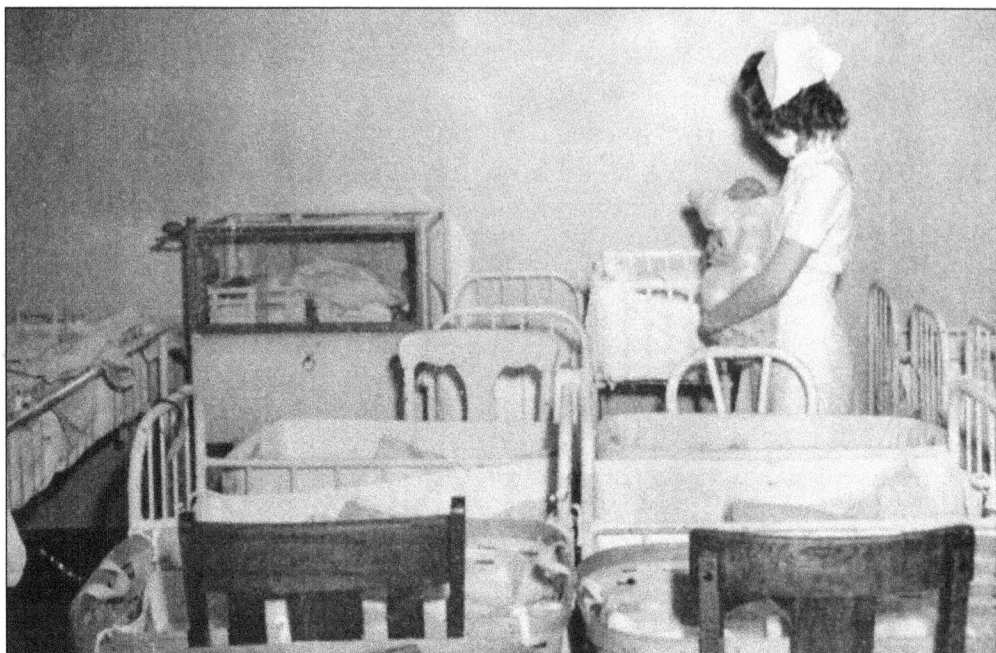

Images of the overcrowding that prevailed at J. C. Blair in the late 1940s were used to advantage in the campaign for funds to build a large addition. In the nursery, clothes baskets on chairs held the overflow of babies—19 in space intended for 14, but holding as many as 26 on a "bumper day." Nurses in pediatrics had to squeeze between the crammed-together cribs. Facilities had not been expanded since 1911, and hospital personnel were trying to accommodate 3,126 patients in 1946 in quarters that had housed just 331 during 1912. Beds lined the halls, and the maternity department struggled to find places for 552 babies born in 1946, compared to the 313 born just four years earlier. Clearly, something had to be done.

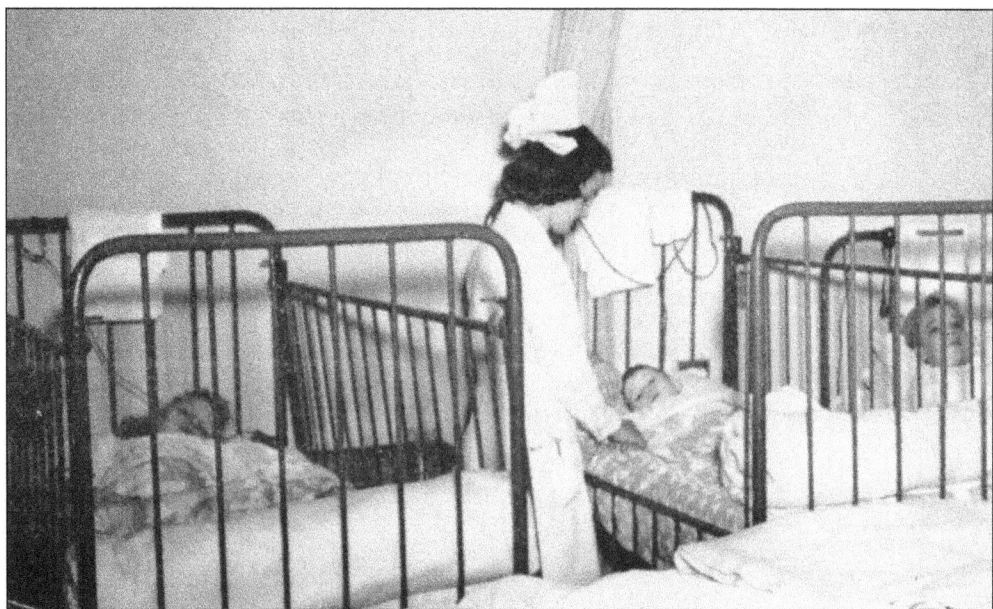

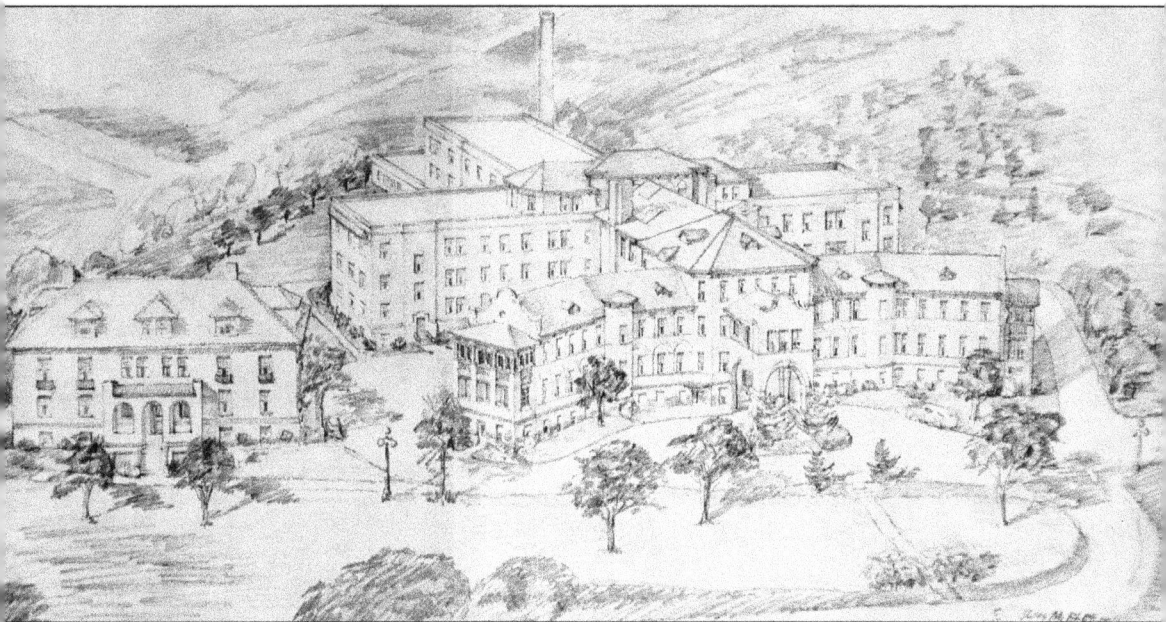

This architect's sketch of the proposed 1950 addition shows that the original Mission Revival style hospital and nurses' residence were to remain the public "face" of the institution. The addition sat behind the original building and was entirely utilitarian in appearance. While the addition's footprint was similar in size to the 1911 structure, it more than doubled that building's capacity. And the standards guiding everything from its operating and emergency departments to its kitchen and laundry facilities reflected 40 years of technological advancement. More doctors practicing locally were sending more patients to the hospital for treatment and keeping them there for an increased number of "patient days"—from 5,971 in 1912 to 29,204 in 1946. More beds were desperately needed.

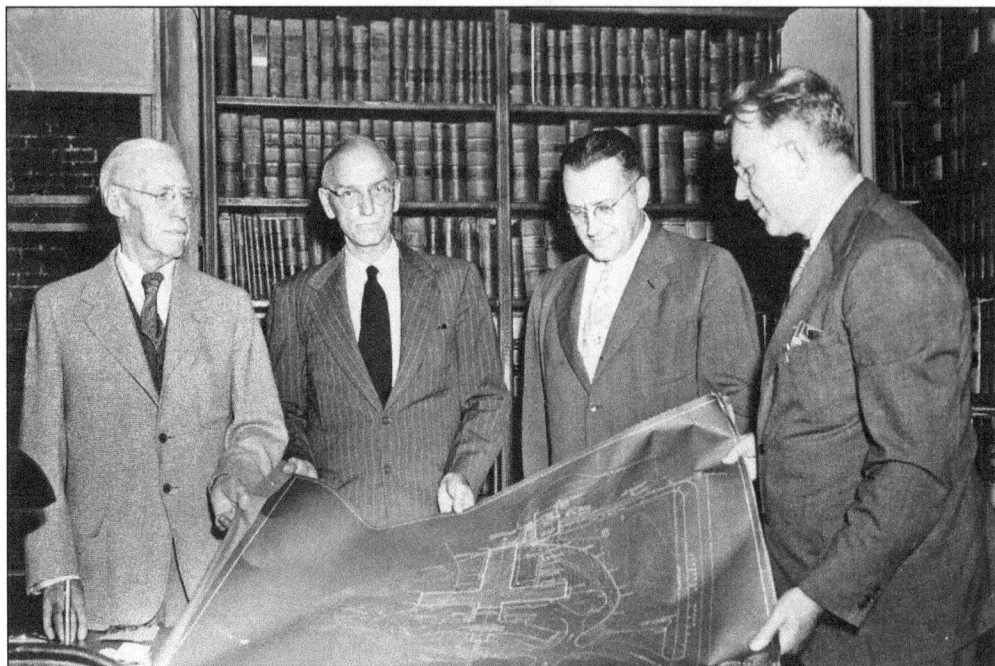

Studying blueprints for the 1950 addition to the hospital are, from left to right, Thomas F. Bailey, longtime board president; E. B. Africa, building committee chairman; Leon Houck, hospital administrator; and a representative of the architects Chatfield and Schlicher, Philadelphia. At ground breaking ceremonies for the project on June 26, 1949, Judge Bailey had the honor of turning the first spade of earth for the $1 million building. He died just two weeks later.

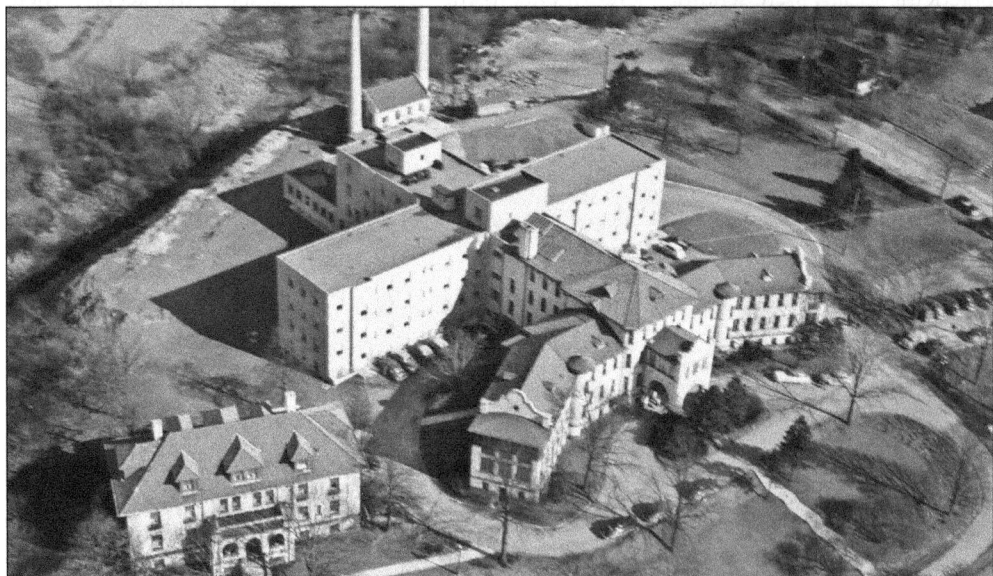

In this aerial image, photographer Lewis Greene chose the perfect angle of the sun and the airplane to highlight the 1950 addition. Also clearly visible are the areas where the county nursing home would join the west end of the new building to the former nurses' residence, and the Acute Care Wing would join the east ends of the 1911 and 1950 buildings. (Courtesy of Isett Acres Museum.)

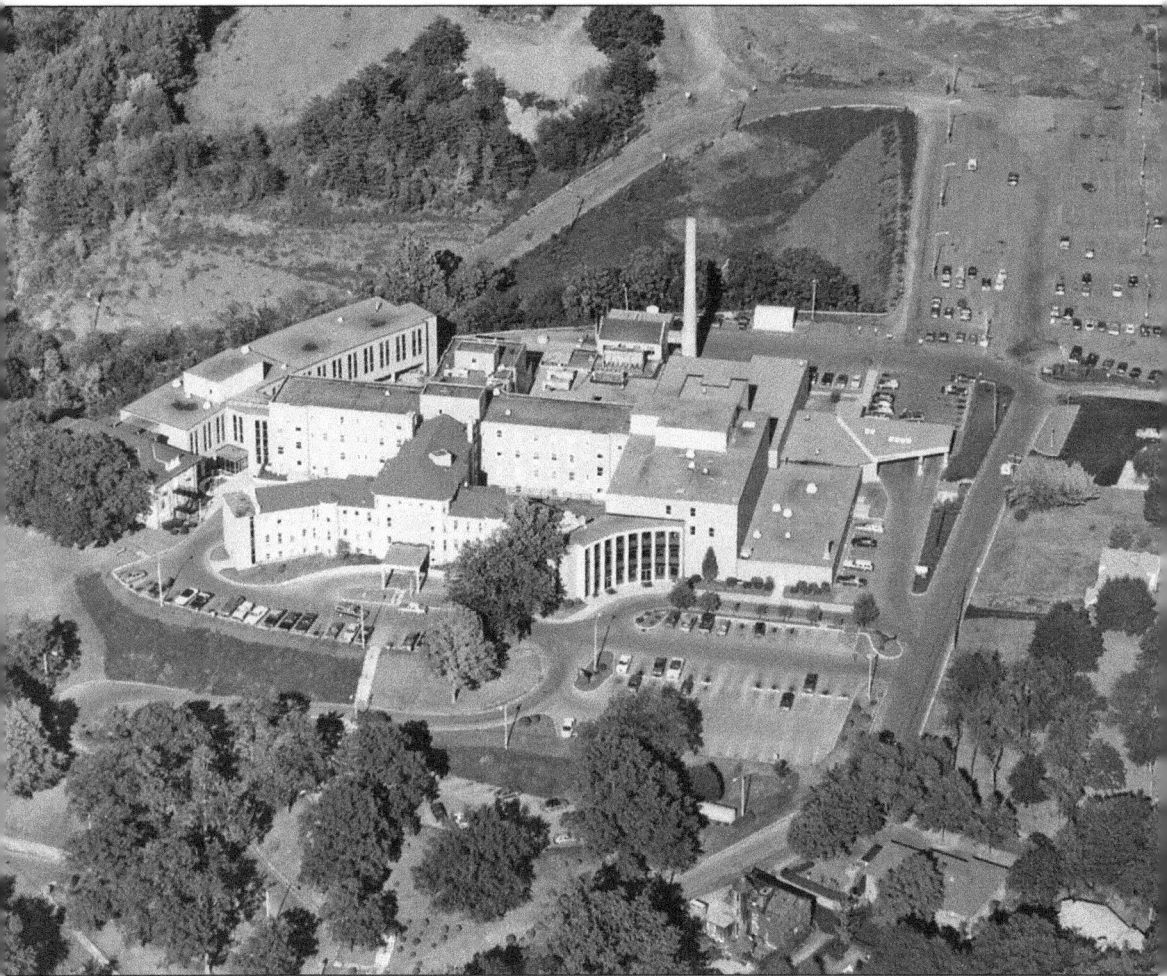

This later aerial view provides an overview of what the 1970–1972 projects in the hospital's $2.97 million expansion looked like. At the west end of the 1950 building is the new county nursing home, which also links to the former nurses' residence. The east ends of the 1911 and 1950 buildings are joined by the new Acute Care Wing. The 1911 building's entrance pavilion and porte cochere have been replaced by a modern covered entrance. The original hospital and the former nurses' residence now held doctors' offices; all hospital functions had been moved to the newer buildings. Huntingdon County had been mandated to provide nursing home services for county residents. The facility was built for $1.76 million by the county and operated by the hospital. It was later sold to a private company.

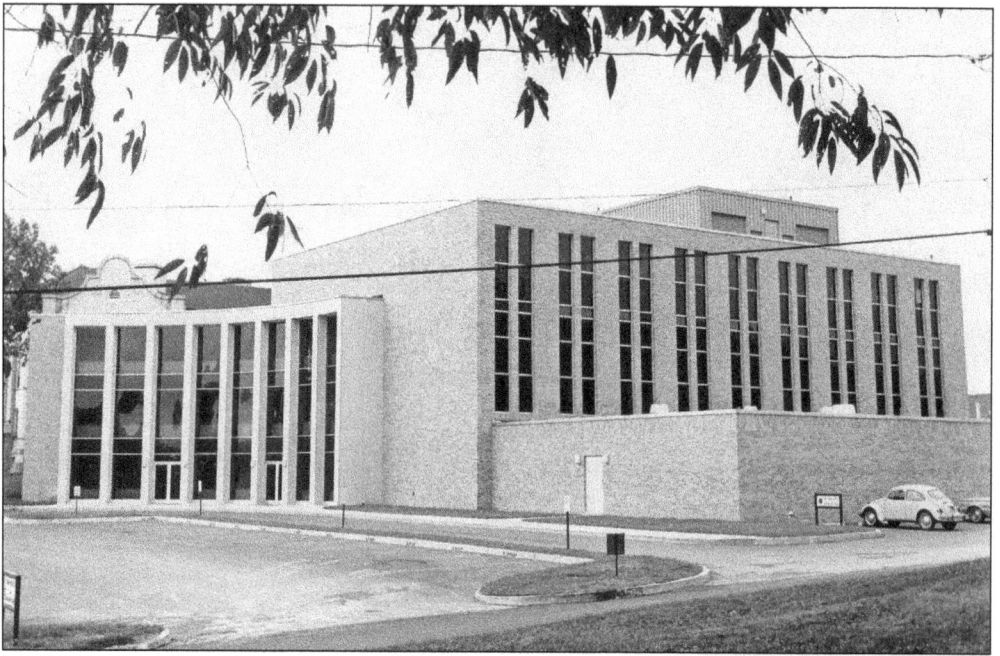

The gable end of the 1911 building can be seen above the left side of the hospital's new main entrance. The Acute Care Wing's curved facade made linking to the original curved structure possible. The new wing contained the emergency/outpatient department, radiology, physical therapy, pediatrics, and the intensive-coronary care unit.

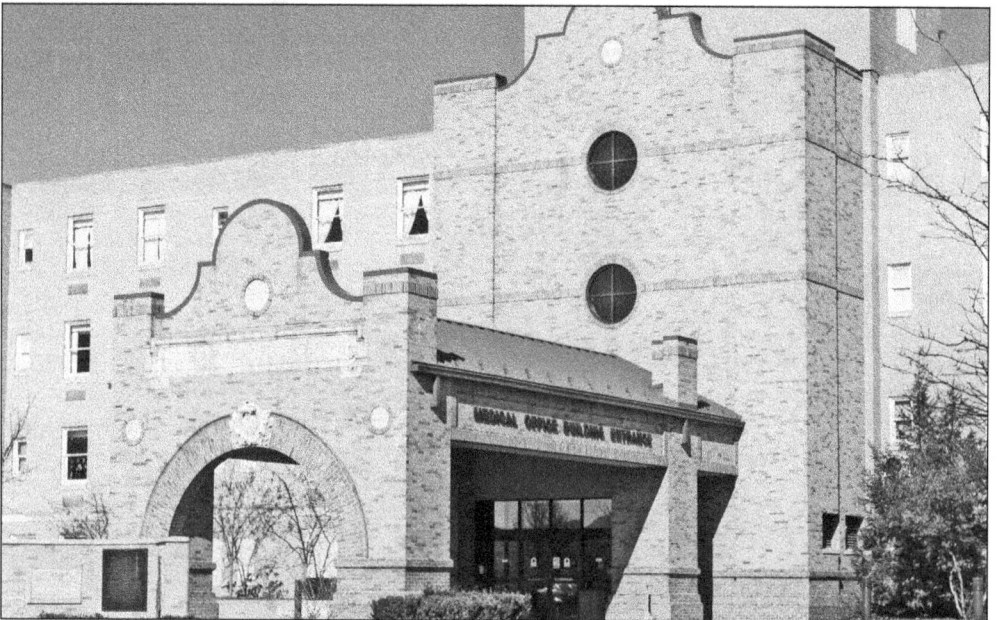

In late 1991, following serious deliberation, the trustees announced their intention to demolish the 1911 building, patiently explaining the financial considerations and code issues driving the decision. Demolition took place in 1996. The new entrance designed for the 1950 building recalls elements of the original structure and includes the name and cartouche saved from the porte cochere.

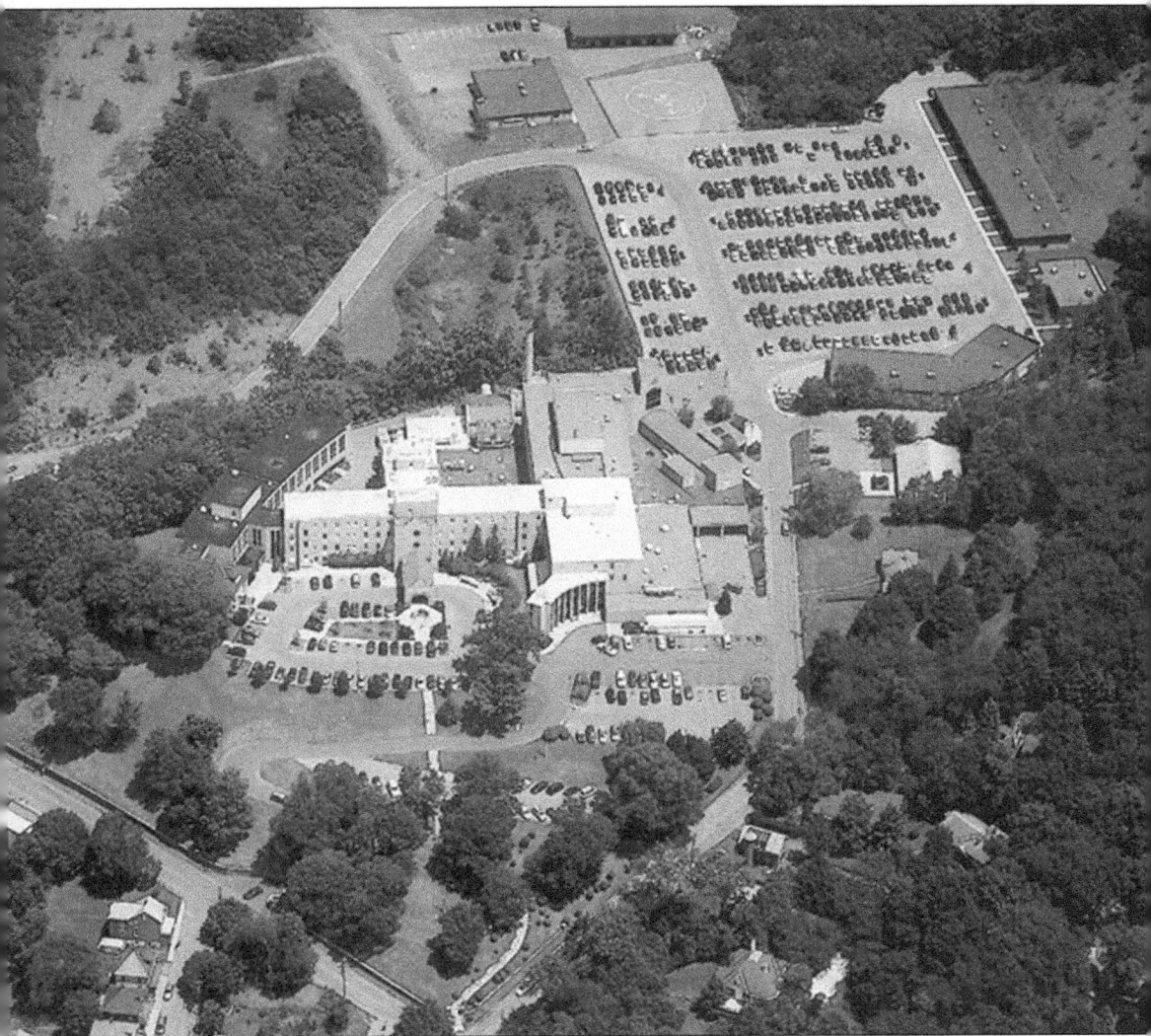

In this 2002 aerial view of the hospital complex, only the winding drive and the endless steps remain of the institution's original site plan. Construction projects during the 1980s and 1990s added classroom and office buildings on the perimeter of the parking area, a separate physical therapy building near the rear of the lot, and a heliport. A new access road from Fourteenth and Warm Springs Avenue provided an alternative to both the winding drive and the steep yellow brick hill. This approach called for a new main entrance, oriented in the direction from which most patients, visitors, and employees would now arrive at the hospital.

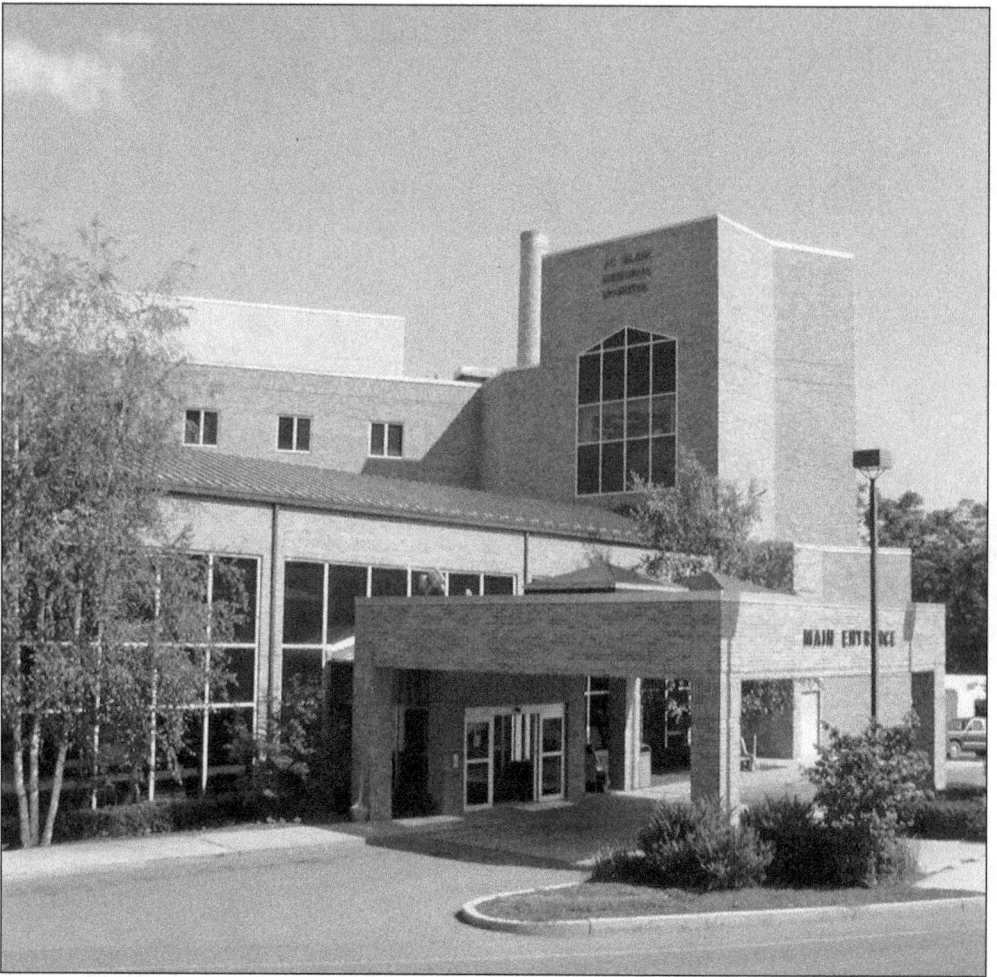

J. C. Blair Memorial Hospital's new main entrance invites comparison with its original entrance. Both recognized the desirability of a covered entranceway, to provide protection from inclement weather. Both had vestibules to keep blasts of cold air out. But the old building had six or eight steps to climb, while the new entrance features automatic doors and ground-level access that wheelchairs or those on foot can easily negotiate. Inside, four registration cubicles for processing the paperwork of those coming for outpatient procedures are reminders that more people using the hospital today are outpatients than are admitted. In Blair Hospital's most recent year, only 2,935 patients were admitted, while 336,120 laboratory tests and 48,739 radiology procedures were performed, the majority of them for outpatients.

Seven

EMERGENCIES

The Pennsylvania Limited No. 2 was approaching Warrior Ridge, west of Huntingdon; running late, the engineer was trying to gain time. The train, consisting of 11 cars, including diners and Pullmans, was nearing its date with destiny.

Tragedy struck just after 11:00 a.m., February 15, 1912, when a coupling came undone and 10 cars jumped the track, plunging 20 feet down the embankment. Three people died on impact; 42 passengers and 25 railroad employees were injured. And five-month-old J. C. Blair Memorial Hospital was pitched headlong into its first major emergency.

Being prepared for the unexpected and knowing how to respond is one of a hospital's ever-present responsibilities. Blair Hospital responded "nobly," in the words of the *Local News*, to its first trial, and has demonstrated its readiness in every emergency since that time. Through the century, various initiatives have addressed the hospital's ability to cope with emergency situations.

In the 1930s, hospital supervisor Helen Stabler appealed to the trustees to establish an accident ward and to the Auxiliary to equip it. Both responded favorably, and the foundation for what became the Emergency Department was laid. The need she identified has multiplied exponentially over the years. The expansion of emergency services and facilities has been part of almost every construction project, and the challenge of staffing this department has repeatedly demanded attention.

In a related initiative, incorporating an intensive care unit into the hospital facilities answered a need to more closely monitor certain patients. Originally a coronary unit, its purpose has been expanded to include other life-threatening conditions—thus, its current designation as an Intensive Critical Care Unit.

Regular drills to practice for emergencies keep hospital personnel's responses sharp. And the surrounding communities raise funds for up-to-date ambulances and trained emergency personnel to man them. Preparedness is still the key word—at J. C. Blair and in the larger community.

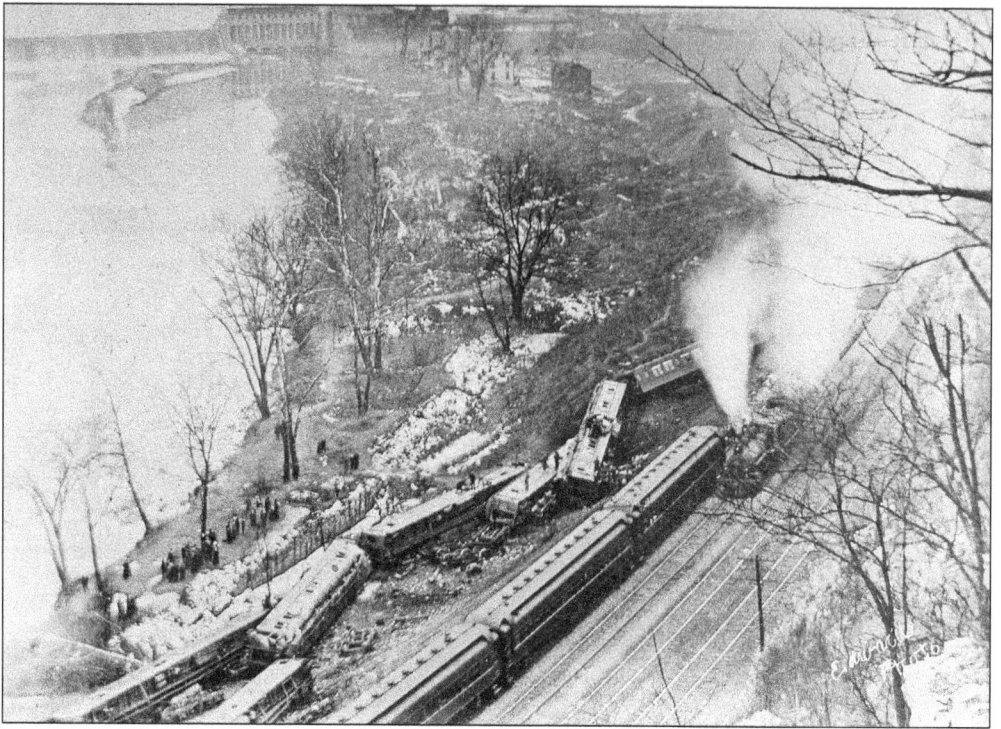

The afternoon sun shone down upon these twisted, dented railroad cars lying on their sides along the Juniata River, below the Warrior Ridge dam. Special trains brought doctors and nurses to help at J. C. Blair Memorial Hospital, which treated 51 victims of the tragic wreck. Ten others received care at the Leister House until beds could be found for them.

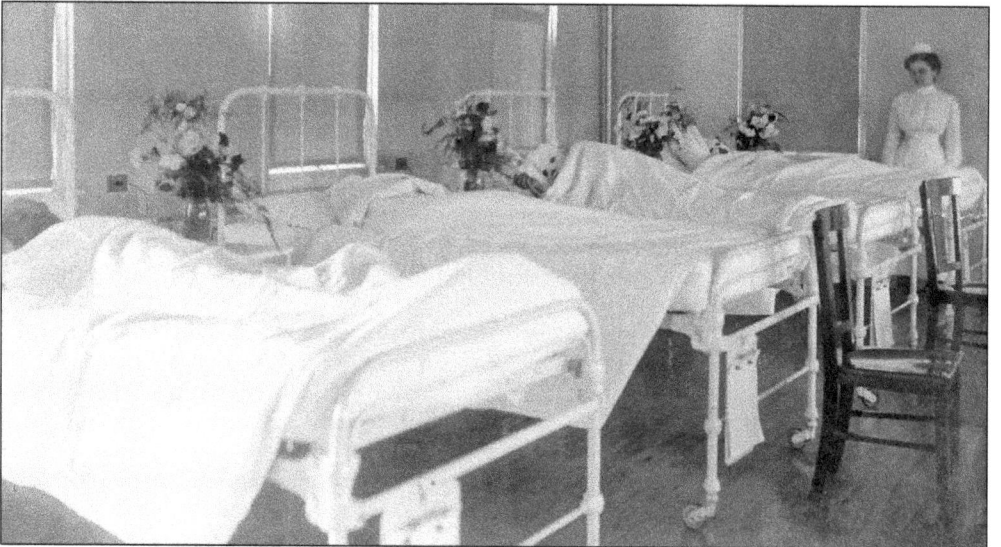

Some of the kitchen and dining car personnel were horribly burned when a stove exploded, scalding them with boiling water. The men seen here with bandaged faces were likely among them. Four of those burned died of their injuries. The Pennsylvania Railroad sent flowers and offered extra beds and linens. Superintendent Pena Schneider refused them, saying, "We have everything we need."

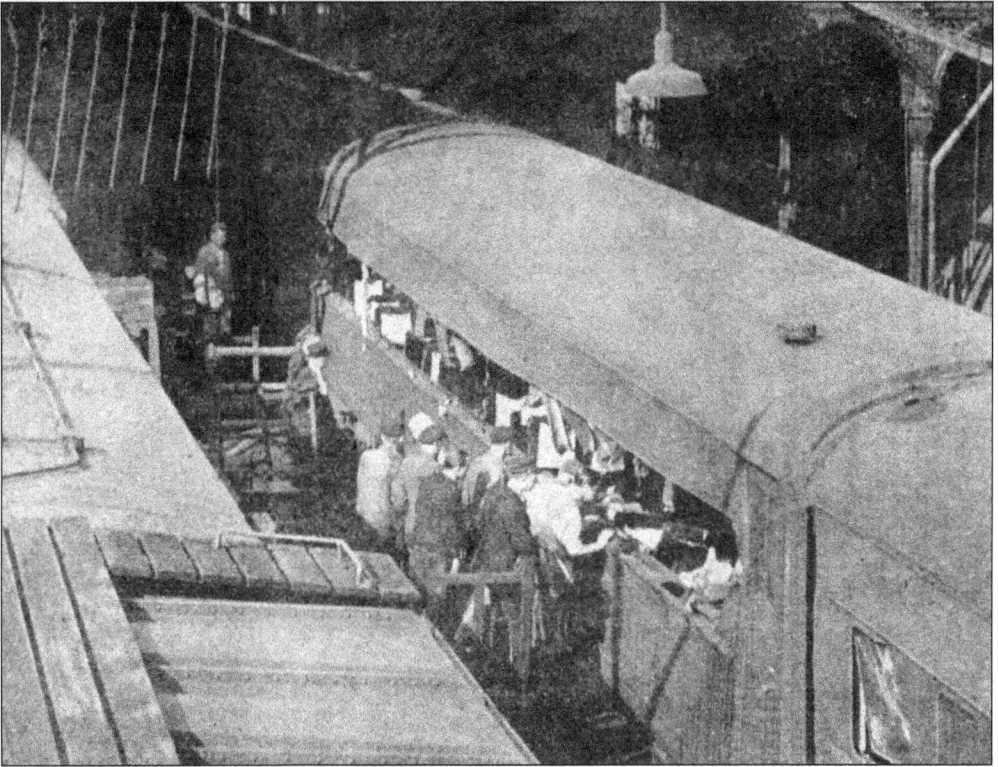

A train wreck on May 1, 1947, happened on a curve east of Petersburg. A 1-inch thick steel plate, 16 feet long by 10.5 feet wide, shifted position on a passing freight train, slicing into the side of a passenger coach on the American Express. Five died and 46 were injured in the worst railroad accident in this area in many years.

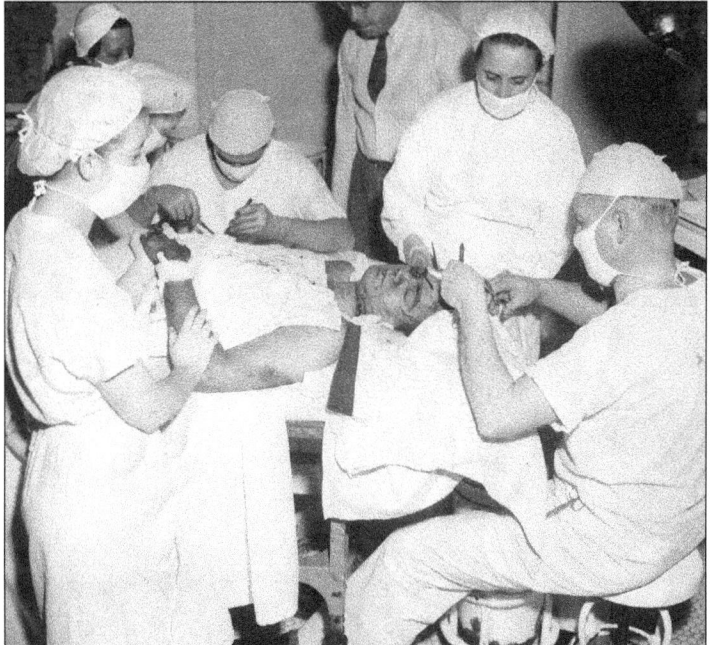

Drs. John B. Fillman (seated center), H. Ford Clark (plain clothes), and Frederic H. Steele (far right) attended to Joseph P. Monaco's injuries, assisted by nurses Jane Guerin, Mrs. Scheffler, Jane Newton, and Jeannette Schell. Judge Thomas F. Bailey told *The Daily News*: "This terrible disaster, with its large number of seriously injured men, women and children, dramatizes better than words possibly could, the great need for increased facilities at the hospital."

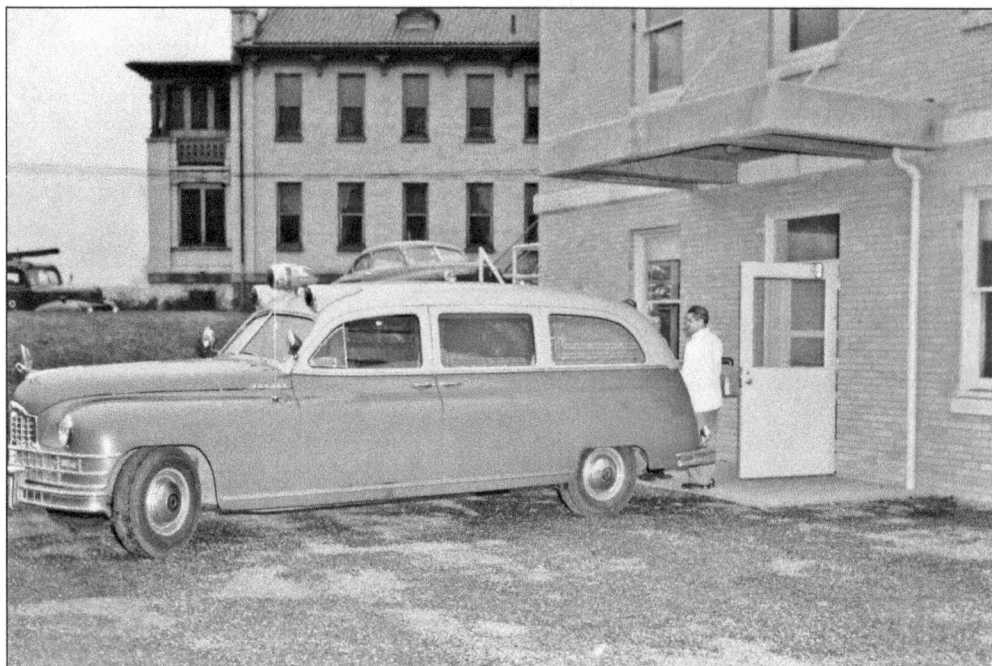

Ambulances of various types have carried patients to the hospital since its beginning. The hospital's first horse-drawn ambulance was succeeded by motorized ambulances, purchased in 1914 and 1928. Later the tradition of fire or ambulance company ownership began. An even greater change occurred when ambulances evolved from simply transporting patients to providing emergency medical technicians (EMT) to care for patients while en route to the hospital. This 1948 Henney model Packard ambulance delivered patients to the emergency room door, where the staff waited to render assistance. Below, during one of the drills conducted periodically to prepare hospital employees to deal with actual disasters, a 1956 Cadillac ambulance and a fire company ladder truck were used to evacuate patients. The highlight of this 1962 exercise was the ladder truck's ability to reach patients on the upper floors of the hospital.

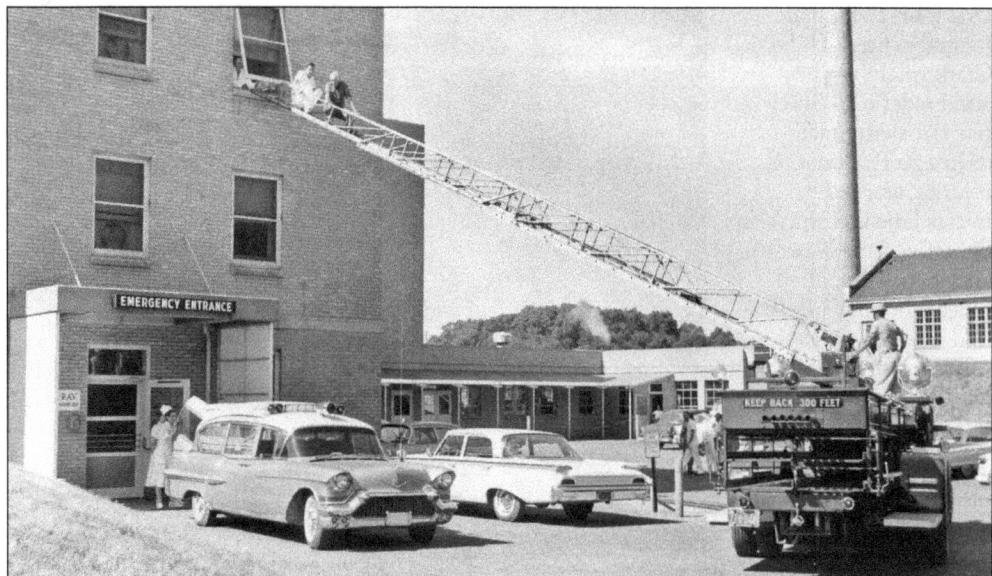

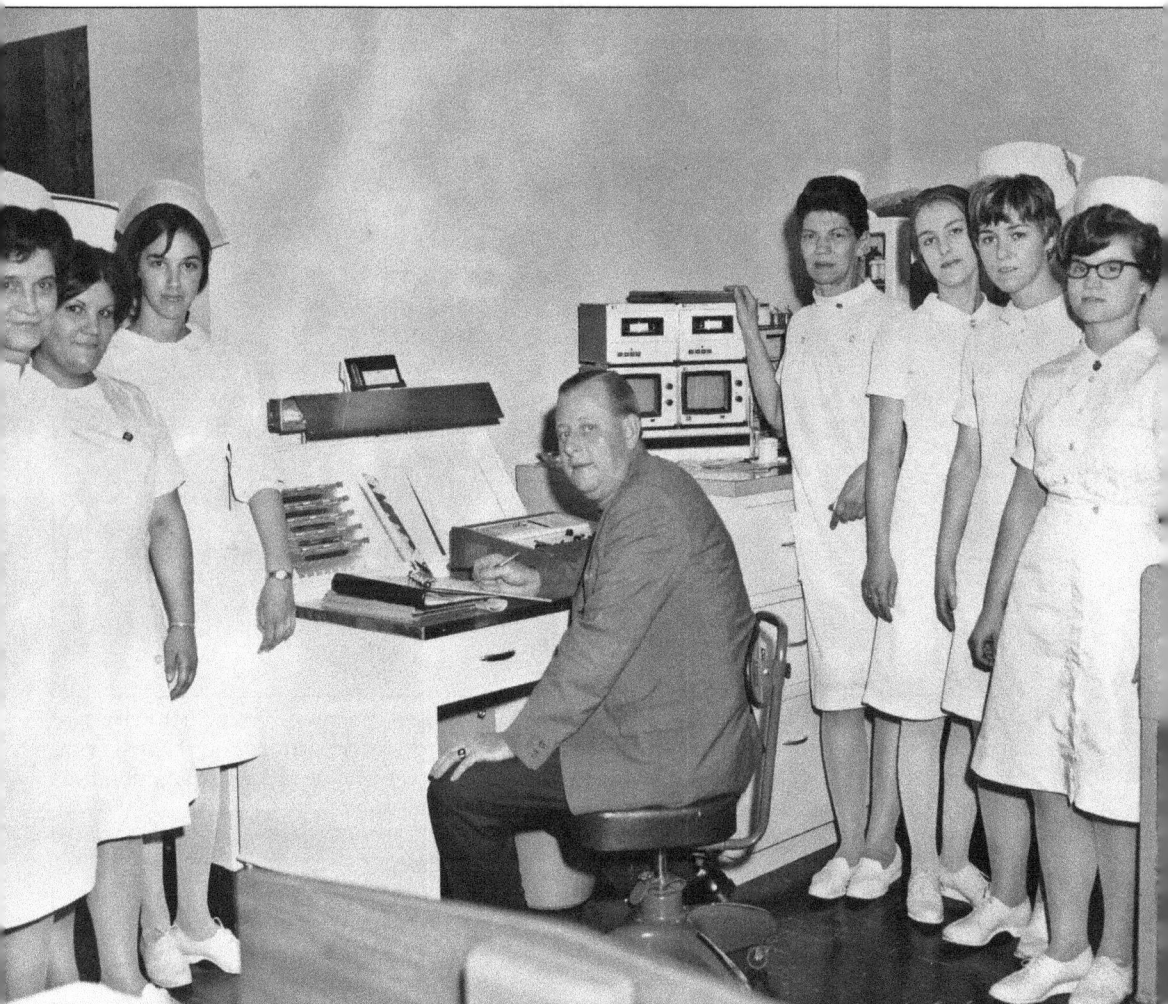

Early in 1970, the hospital launched a new program when Dr. H. William Stewart was designated the first emergency room physician. Prior to his appointment, staff doctors were "on call" on a rotating basis. Here Stewart posed with his staff. From left to right are director of nurses Pauline Barry, Salina Kanagy, Mary Casselberry, Dorothy Adams, Vicky Shope, Linda Holland, and Charlotte Hostetler. In his new position, Stewart worked from 12 noon until 12 midnight, four days a week, with staff doctors filling in as needed. A Huntingdon native and Juniata College graduate, Stewart was a 1945 Jefferson Medical College graduate and completed a one-year surgical residency. He had also served two years in the Army Medical Corps during World War II. In 1948, after working at the hospital with Dr. Francis S. Mainzer, he opened a private practice in Alexandria.

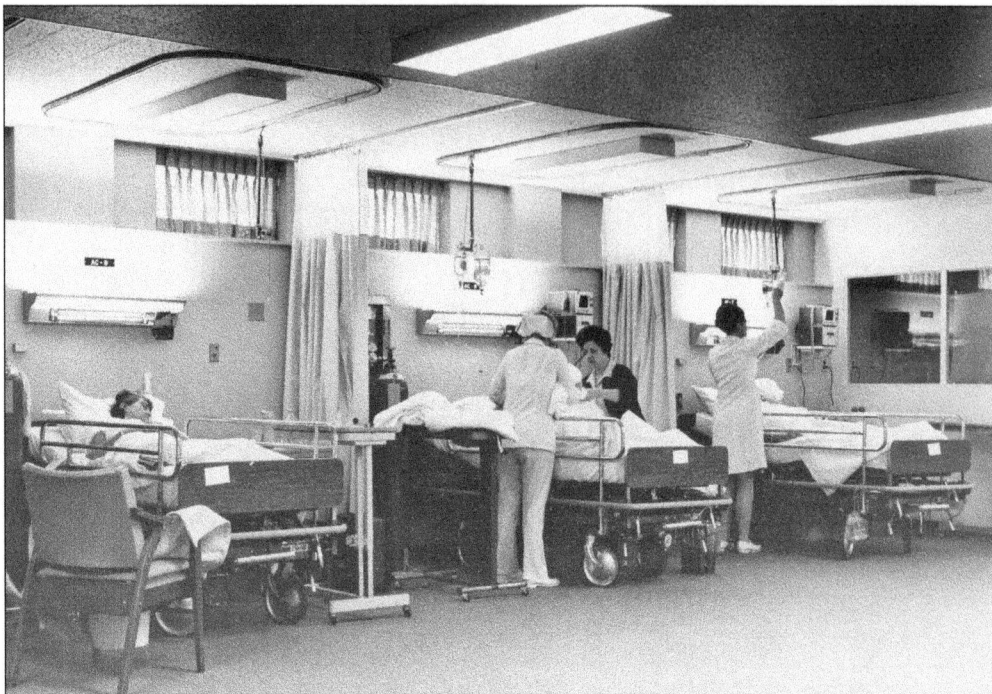

When the Acute Care Wing was completed in 1972, it housed the intensive and coronary care unit on the second floor, as well as the new emergency/outpatient department on the first floor. The rising utilization of emergency services, which had driven the need for the addition, was reported to have increased by 300 percent in just the past few years.

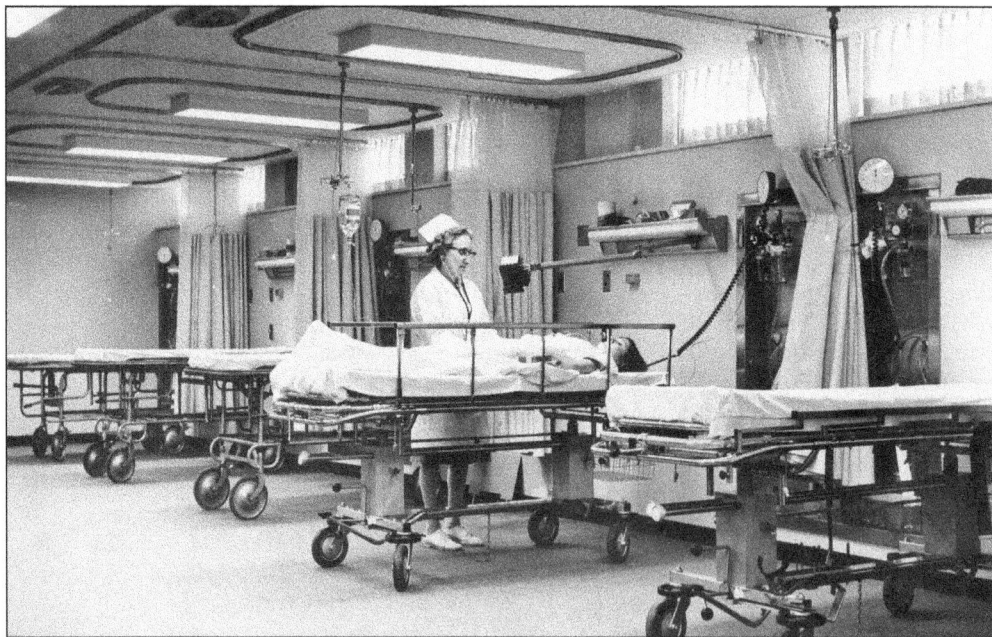

Jeannette Schell was in charge of the new recovery room facilities in the Acute Care Wing. An experienced nurse and J. C. Blair graduate, she had worked in a similar position since the opening of the hospital's first recovery room in 1955.

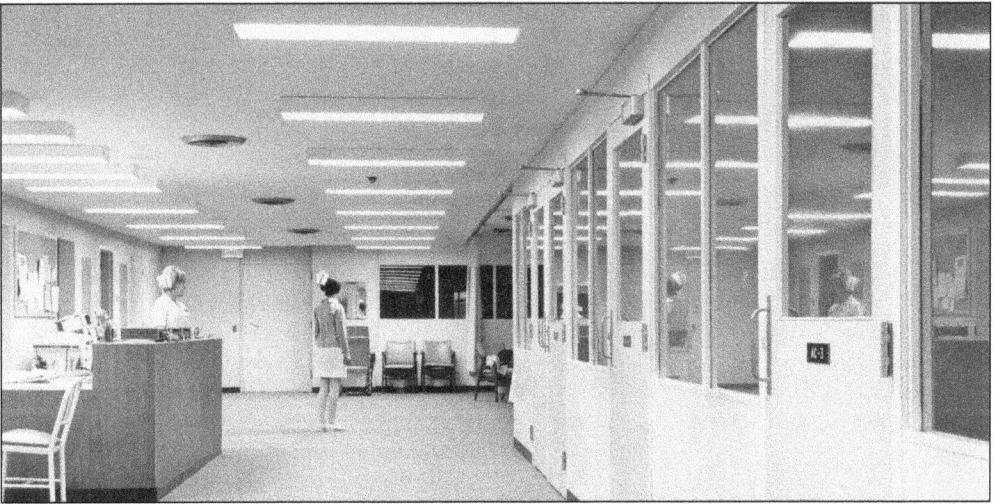

Five registered nurses completed six months of training for work in the new intensive and coronary care unit seen above. The course was taught by Del Kowalski, seen below (left) with Dr. Robert H. Beck, chairman of the intensive and coronary care committee, as he awarded certificates to, from left to right, Linda A. Baker, Darlene K. Brosius, Marsha L. Schreiber, and Glenda K. Hartzler. Barbara Fleck Wright was not present for the photograph on August 27, 1972. The nurses learned to read cardiac monitoring equipment, recognize cardiac arrhythmias, and use emergency measures, such as defibrillation and heart massage. Dr. Beck declared, "These nurses have successfully completed a difficult and sophisticated course of instruction and training in intensive and coronary care nursing. The graduates of this course are now fully qualified to work in the hospital's intensive and coronary care unit, and we are very proud of them."

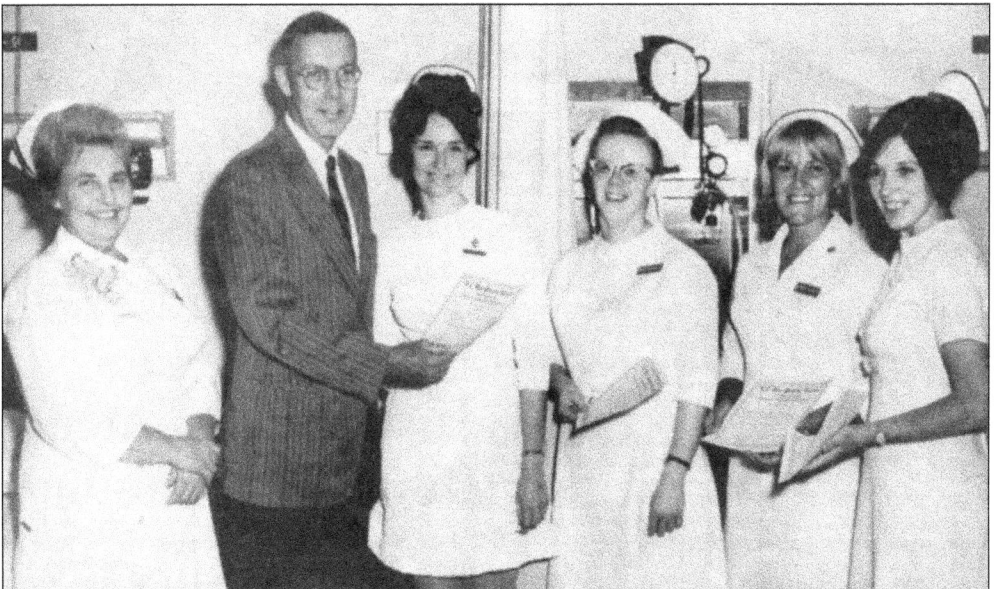

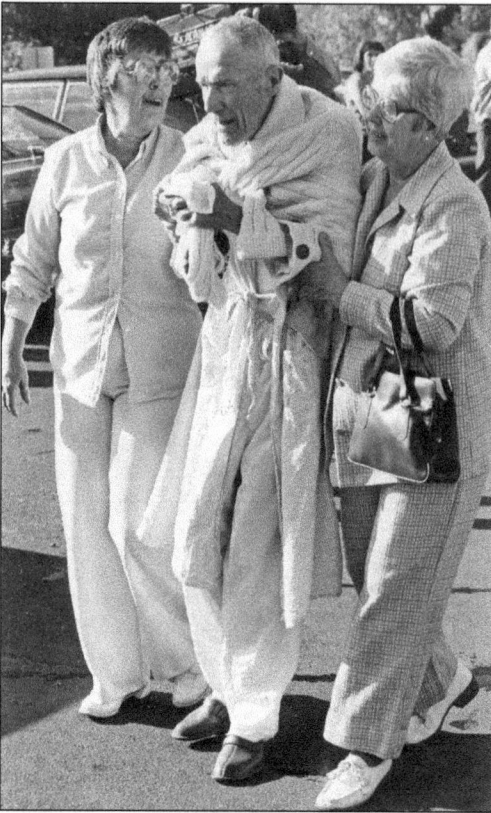

It was not a fire drill when the alarm sounded at 4:12 on the afternoon of October 9, 1981—it was a real emergency! A construction worker's torch accidentally ignited ceiling insulation in the basement. Acrid smoke quickly spread throughout the hospital. But all the years of practice had prepared the staff well, and everyone quickly stepped into action. Help came from a seven-county area as volunteer ambulance crews and paramedics hurried to the scene. Working together, they evacuated all 86 patients. Some were moved into the adjoining County Nursing Home; others were transferred to hospitals in the area or discharged to their own homes. After eight days of cleaning and preparation, the hospital reopened for business as usual on October 17.

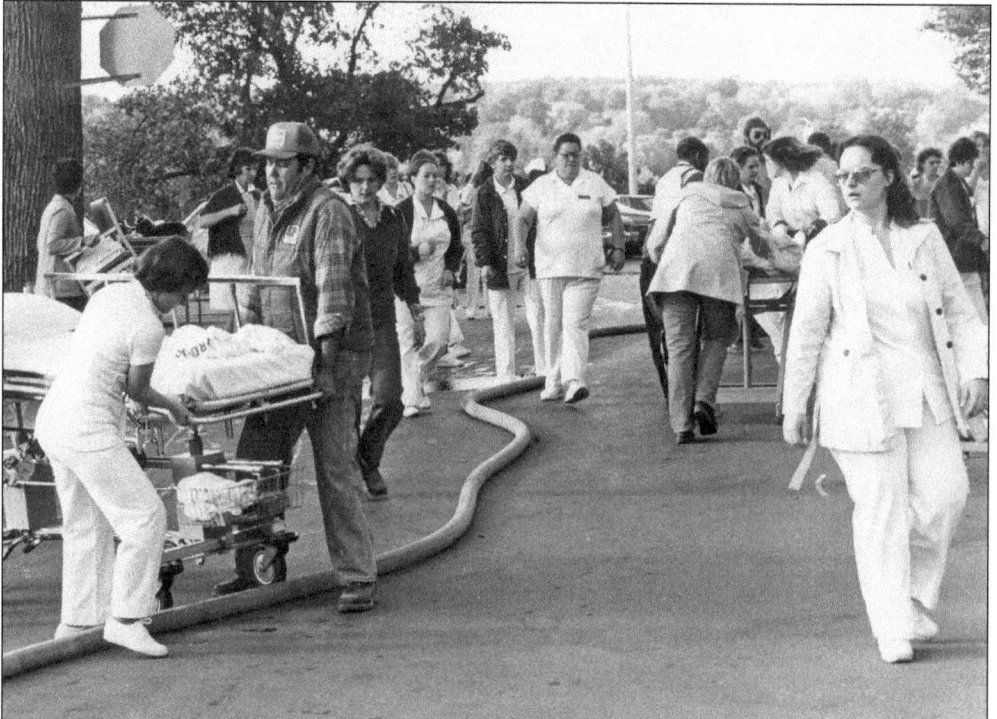

Eight

CHANGING TIMES

Like transportation and communication, medicine and medical technology have been transformed over the past century by remarkable inventions and scientific advances. The diagnostic technologies available to physicians and their patients today would have amazed the doctors practicing when J. C. Blair Memorial Hospital opened in 1911, as would the medications, laboratory procedures, surgical techniques, and treatment options that doctors can employ to extend life and to cure many ills for which there used to be no cure.

The folksy, horse-and-buggy doctor in a Norman Rockwell painting is certainly viewed through a rosy haze, but there is no doubt that doctor-patient relationships are different when a family's care is divided among numerous specialists who treat different ages, different sexes, and different organs and systems of the body. Yet few patients would trade the modern drugs, diagnostic procedures, and advanced treatments they are offered today for the old-fashioned, kindly doctor whose best treatment option was often to hold a patient's hand and hope his body was strong enough to overcome whatever afflicted him.

One of the century's dramatic changes is the cost of utilizing all these advances in medical treatment and technology. What has not changed is many patients' inability to pay these costs. Many were unable to pay even the low fees charged in the hospital's early days. The hospital ran a deficit regularly in its early history, and that, unfortunately, has often been Blair Hospital's plight in later years, as well.

Over the years, the hospital has broadened its mission, especially in the realm of outreach programs that promote healthy living. School instruction, expectant parent classes, and sessions for women on their special health concerns advocate for awareness and knowledge as tools for staying healthy and preventing illness and disease, rather than being treated after one's health has been compromised.

Making modern medicine and medical technology available to the community, and making the community aware of the tools at hand for living longer and better, continues to be the mission of J. C. Blair Memorial Hospital, however the times may change.

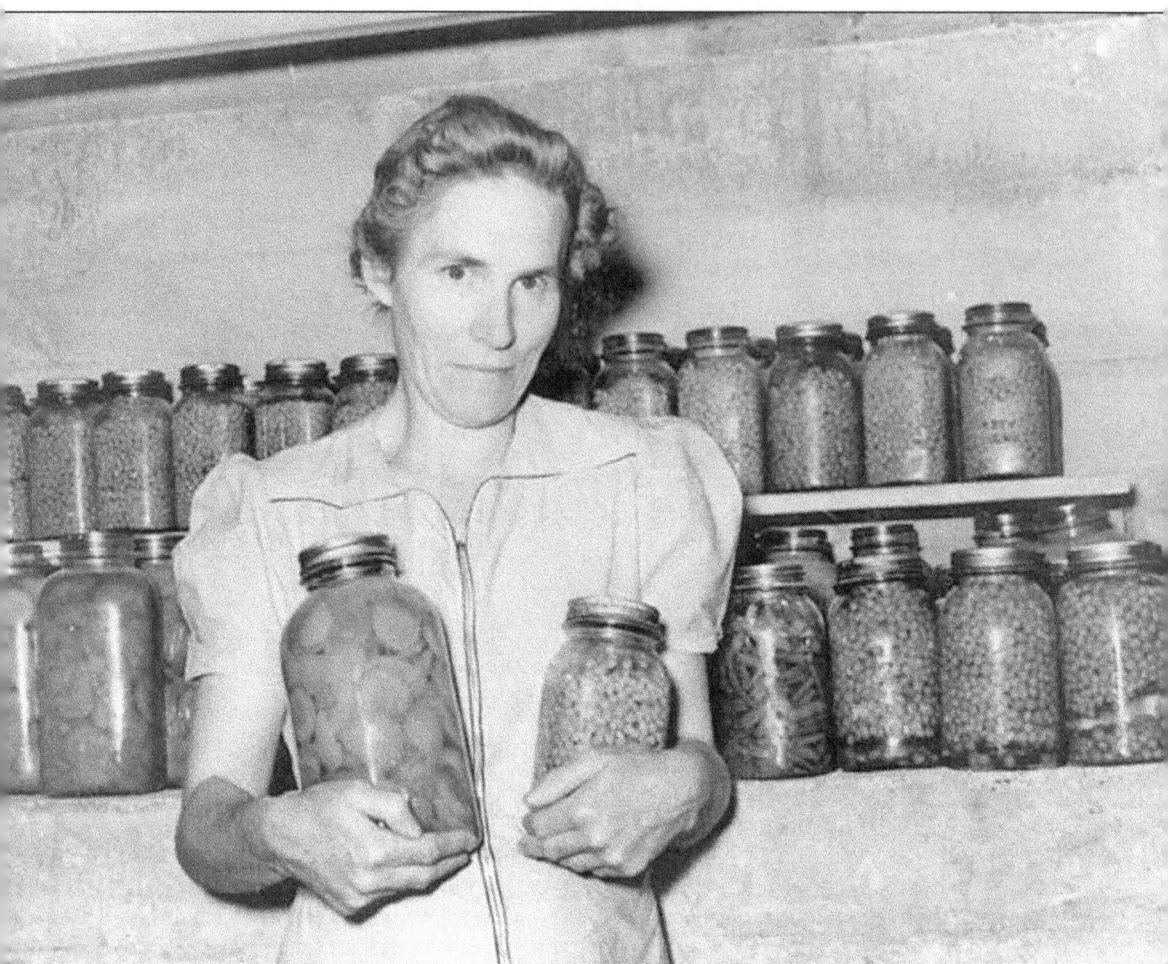

This woman may be selecting home-canned fruits and vegetables to contribute to one of J. C. Blair Memorial Hospital's annual donation days. Today rules governing where and how food is prepared would not permit such a practice, and regulation is probably what put an end to the popular donation program. A five-page list of what the community donated, published in the 1918 annual report, includes a case of whiskey from Martin Grube, four dozen bottles of soda from H. D. Reiners, 100 pounds of flour from Hellyer's Mill, 34 quarts of cherries from a single donor, every kind of canned fruit and jelly imaginable, a few cans of tuna fish and lobster, potatoes, sweet potatoes, cabbage, pumpkins, apples, pears, plums, grapes, crates of oranges and grapefruit, gallons of apple butter, eggs, chili sauce, canned tomatoes, flour, cornmeal, sugar, salt, coffee, cocoa, molasses, syrup, honey, milk, grape juice, wine, napkins, towels, soap, nightgowns, kimonos, muslin, magazines, books, some lightly used clothing, and a few chickens and deer.

No. _____ C. No. _____ HUNTINGDON, PA., *March 16,* 193*1*

MR. *Harry Grubb*

IN ACCOUNT WITH J. C. BLAIR MEMORIAL HOSPITAL

BILLS PAYABLE WEEKLY

PRIVATE ROOM	*47* DAYS AT $*5*⁰⁰ PER *day*	*235* —
PRIVATE WARD	*17* " " *3*⁵⁰ " *day*	*59* 50
WARD		
SPECIAL NURSE *Board 2* " *1*⁰⁰ *night*		*2* —
" " BOARD *2* " *1*⁵⁰ " *day*		*3* —
OPERATING ROOM ✓		*5* —
ANESTHETIC ✓		*7* 50
SUPPORTERS		
AMBULANCE ✓		*7* —
DRUGS		
TELEPHONE CALLS		
LABORATORY ✓		*11* —
X-RAY ✓		*50* —
LAUNDRY		*380* —

RECEIVED PAYMENT

_____ SUP'T.

In 21 years, from deep in the Depression to the post-World War II recovery period, the rate for a room at J. C. Blair rose only $3, the operating room charge $5, and the cost of anesthesia remained the same. In 1966, administrator Richard Cummings expressed grave concern over rising hospital costs, which had more than doubled over the past decade, from an average daily cost per patient of $15.56 to $32.23. But the national average of $44.48 made Blair's rise look small by comparison. Causes were attributed to the inclusion of hospital employees in Federal minimum wage legislation and nurses' demands for higher wages. Cummings pronounced the implementation of Medicare less hectic than expected but complained of staggering paperwork and slow reimbursement. All of these familiar concerns are now more than 40 years old.

STATEMENT
J. C. BLAIR MEMORIAL HOSPITAL
HUNTINGTON, PENNSYLVANIA

June 13, 195*2*

*Ernest Stinger
Alexandria, Pa RD #1
Mrs. Kenneth Stinger*

ALL BILLS ARE PAYABLE WEEKLY

BALANCE—Account Rendered		
Room and Board	2 Days @ $ *8.00*	*16.00*
Room and Board	Days @ $	
Operating Room or Delivery Room		*10.00*
Anesthesia		*7.50*
X-ray		
Laboratory		*3.50*
Drugs		*.60*
Special Treatments		
Ambulance		
Telephone		*.06*
Miscellaneous		

RECEIVED PAYMENT
J. C. Blair Memorial Hospital
BY _____ DATE *6/13/52* TOTAL CHARGES *37.66*
For items shown on this statement only
any Additional Charges will be Billed later

TOTAL CREDITS _____

BALANCE — AMOUNT DUE _____

Should this statement be in error, kindly so advise.

111

COMMONWEALTH OF PENNSYLVANIA
DEPARTMENT OF HEALTH

DIPHTHERIA

THESE PREMISES ARE UNDER STATE QUARANTINE

No person shall be permitted to enter, leave or take any article from this house without written permission from a legally authorized agent of the Department of Health, excepting physicians and trained nurses in charge of the sick.

No persons other than those authorized by the Department of Health shall remove this placard. Any person or persons defacing, covering up, or destroying this placard render themselves liable to the penalties of the law.

Act of the General Assembly approved June 28, 1923, provides that anyone violating the provisions of this Act, upon conviction thereof, may be sentenced to pay a fine of not more than $100.00, to be paid to the use of said county, and costs of prosecution, or to be imprisoned in the county jail for a period of not less than ten days or more than thirty days, or both, at the discretion of the court.

By Order of the Department of Health

. . . .
Health Officer

. . . .   Posted 19
Address

Prior to the development of effective vaccines, childhood diseases were widespread, with epidemics occurring annually in many communities. Doctors treated children's symptoms as best they could, and preventive measures were employed to try to contain outbreaks of measles, chicken pox, whooping cough, mumps, or diphtheria. Since the diseases were spread by direct contact with infected persons, quarantining households that had been struck was considered the best method of control. Notices like this were posted conspicuously to alert the public to houses where a contagious disease had been diagnosed, but the signs were often ignored. Many parents preferred that their children contract these diseases and develop immunity while young, as they could be more serious in adulthood. Discovering vaccines that would protect against disease was a long-standing goal of medical research. In the late 1700s, vaccination with cowpox was found to be effective against smallpox. Dr. John Henderson advertised in the Huntingdon *Gazette* in 1801 that he had a supply of "fresh infection" and was prepared to inoculate area citizens. (Courtesy of Dr. James Savory.)

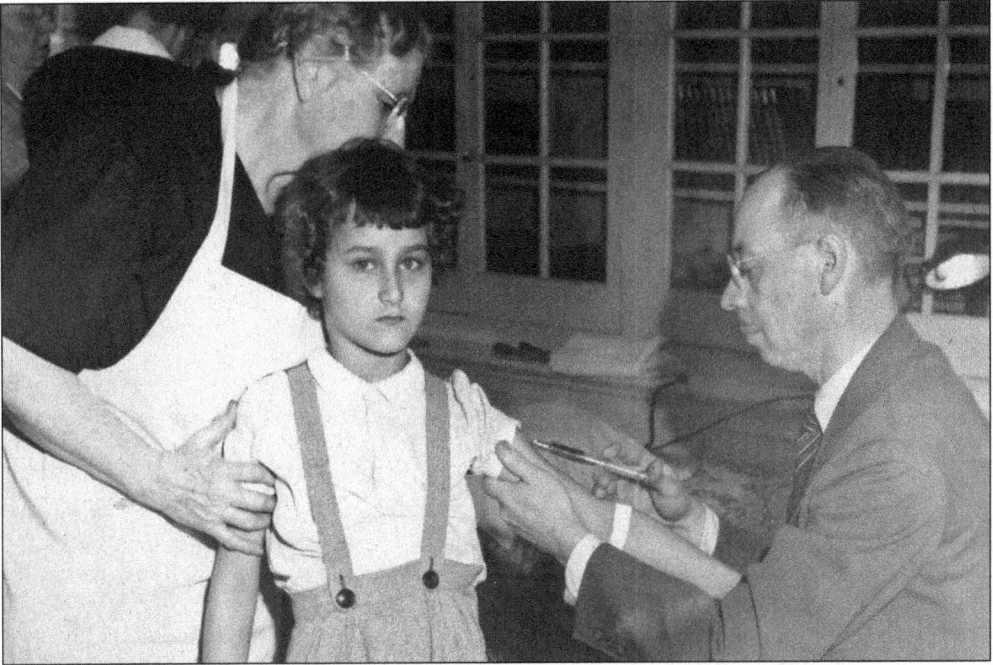

Of all the childhood diseases, polio was the most feared at mid-century because of its crippling effects and possible death. When Dr. Jonas Salk developed an injectable vaccine in 1952, it was eagerly accepted for massive clinical trials in the United States. The results were impressive, although 260 recipients of the "killed" vaccine developed polio and 10 died. (Courtesy of the Pennsylvania Historical and Museum Commission.)

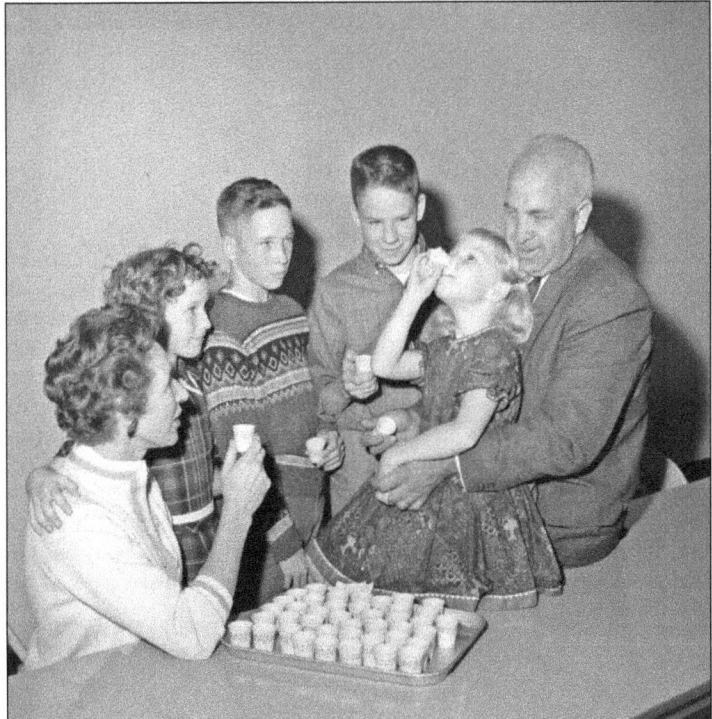

Dr. Albert Sabin developed a "live" polio vaccine that conferred lifelong intestinal, as well as bodily, immunity, ensuring the recipient could not remain a carrier of the disease. Administered on a sugar cube, the vaccine underwent a nationwide trial on Sabin Sunday, October 21, 1962. J. C. Blair's director of nurses, Pauline Barry, oversaw 13 clinics in schools countywide. Here, Hattie LaPorte takes her medicine at Juniata Valley School.

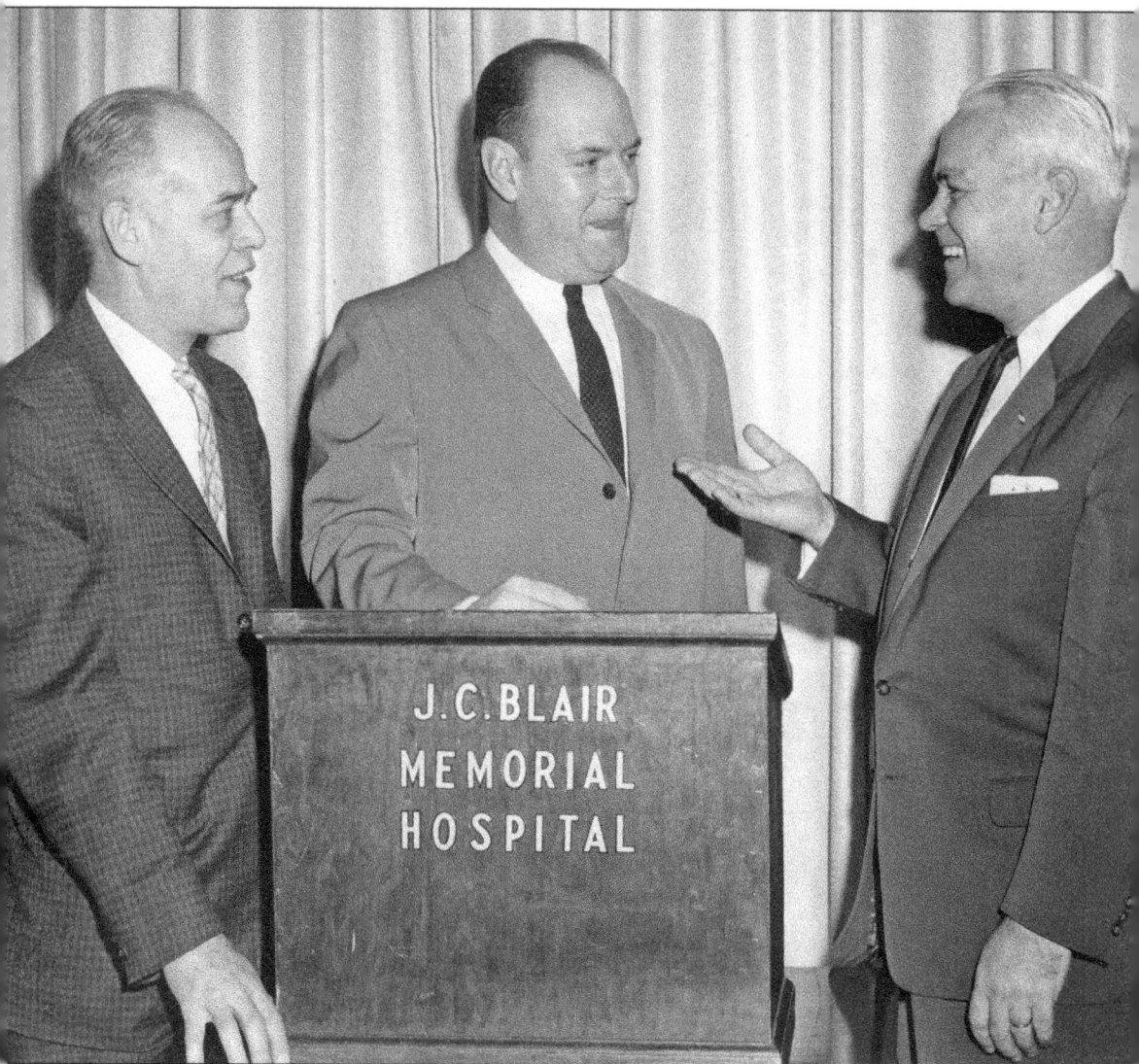

In 1960, Dr. William Patterson (left) and Alva Walton (right), board president, greeted Robert C. Craig, secretary of the Pennsylvania Medical Society's Legislative Committee, who spoke to board members and staff about the Forand Bill. The bill would have provided health insurance to social security beneficiaries. Opposition was successful in keeping the bill from being reported out of committee. Doctors, including the Huntingdon County Medical Society, were long-standing opponents of "socialized medicine," although they did not oppose the state subsidy that J. C. Blair Memorial Hospital received each year in partial support of its care for indigent patients. A Federal subsidy might have helped to reduce the losses incurred by the hospital annually through caring for patients who could not pay. Doctors admitted that care for the elderly was a serious problem, but they hoped to find a way to address it on their own, without government intervention. Just five years later, in 1965, amendments to social security created Medicare, which passed with bipartisan support.

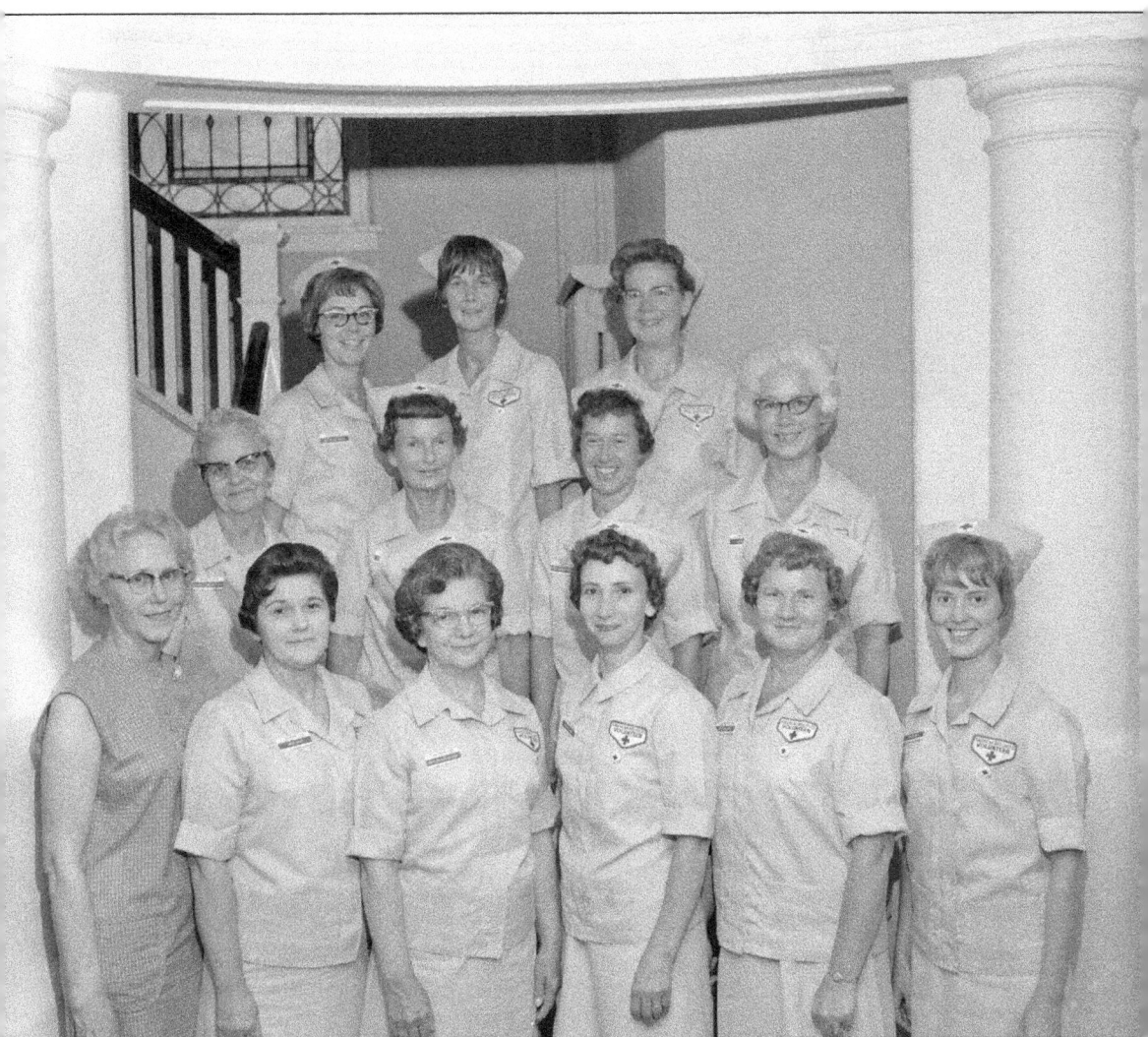

This class of American Red Cross Hospital Volunteers graduated from their training course in June 1967. Red Cross volunteers had already logged 1,325 hours of work in the program, which had begun in January. Shown here, with Elizabeth Bell (left, front), executive director of the local Red Cross chapter, are, from left to right, (first row) Mrs. Paul Cook, Mrs. Earl Householder, Mrs. Blaine Pollock, Mrs. Fay Bryant, and Mrs. William Payne; (second row) Mrs. Clarence Litzenberger, Mrs. Royal Musgrove, Mrs. Harold Hockenberry, and Mrs. John Hanks; (third row) Mrs. Glenn Holsinger, Mrs. Richard Rosenhoover, and Mrs. Dale Hartman. Also graduating, but not present for the photograph, were Mrs. Charles Hoffman, Mrs. Kenneth Kyper, Mrs. George Prendergast, Mrs. Richard Royer, and Mrs. Myron Ulbrich. The Red Cross volunteer program is no longer active at Blair Hospital.

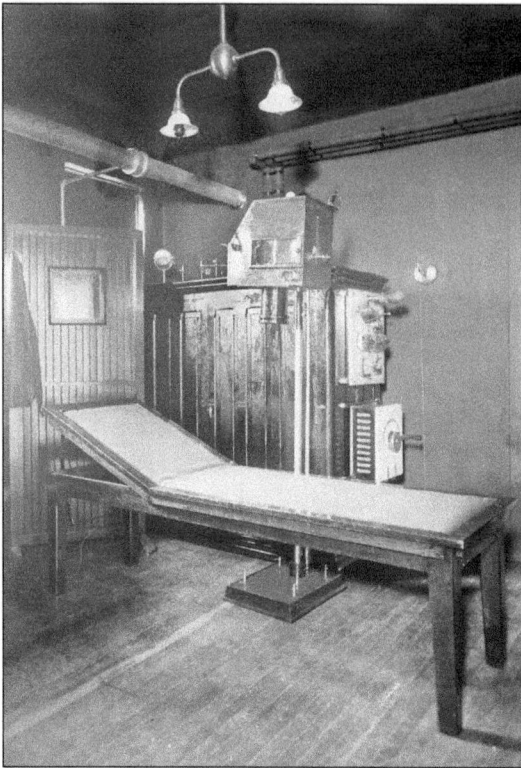

J. C. Blair Memorial Hospital's original x-ray facilities look rather primitive, but since Wilhelm Roentgen's discovery of the x-ray came just 16 years before the hospital opened, hospital planners were actually quite up-to-date in their inclusion of an x-ray department. In charge almost from the beginning, Dr. John M. Keichline headed the department until mid-century.

Blair Hospital's first x-ray tube was a Coolidge tube, like this one. The tubes were developed by William Coolidge, a physicist at General Electric, which manufactured them. Preserved by the hospital as a historical artifact, the tube exhibited a characteristic violet color, indicating the presence of potassium. The fragile tube was broken when it was displayed at the hospital's 75th anniversary celebration. (Photograph by University of Vermont Physics Department.)

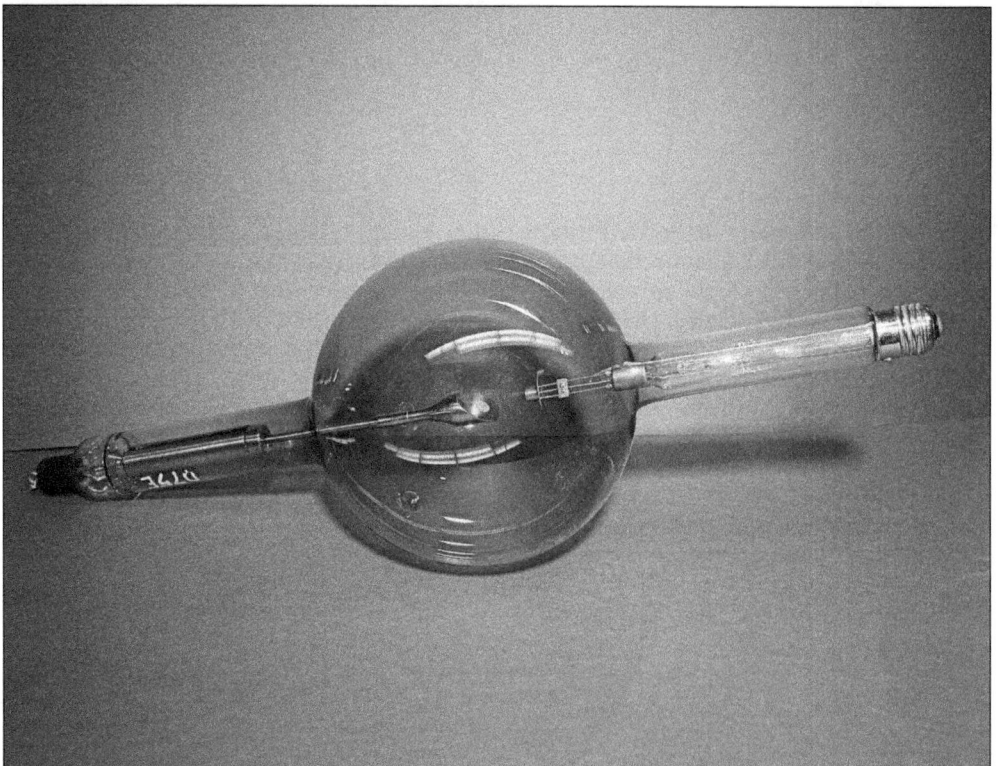

When Dr. Robert Ayella became head of the radiology department, he persuaded five health agencies to share the $12,200 cost of an image intensifier, bringing the department up to the most modern standards. The equipment enabled heart catheterizations to be performed in the region for the first time, a procedure familiar to Ayella and Dr. Burgess Smith. Here Ayella (left) shows Dr. West a new tilting, rotating x-ray table in 1961.

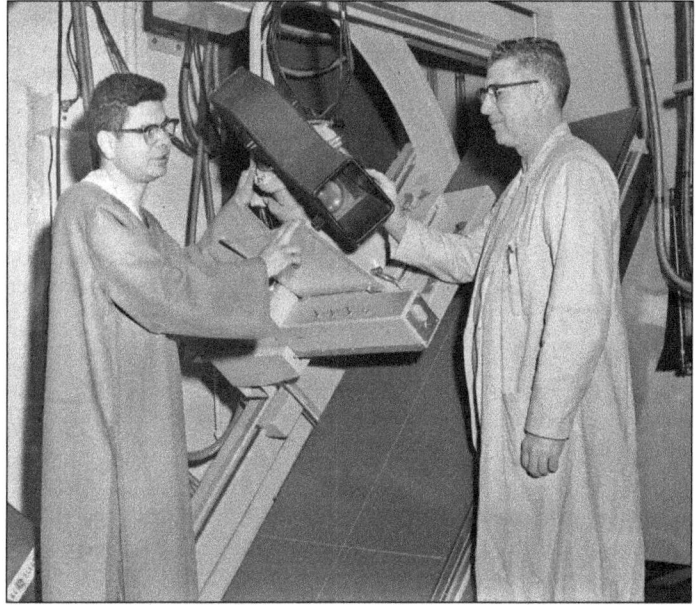

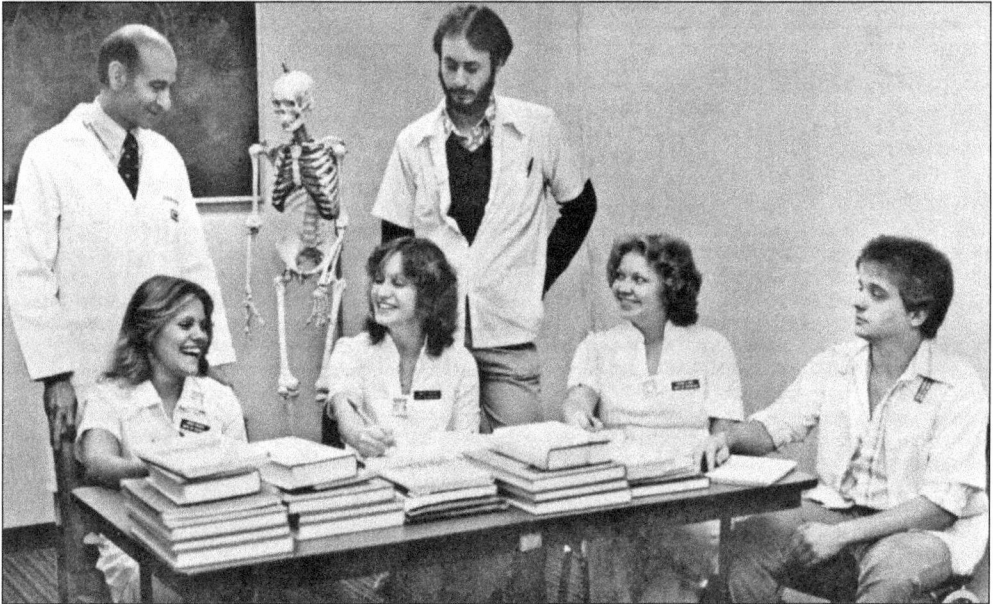

Directed by hospital radiologist Dr. Richard DiDonato (standing, left), an x-ray technology school opened in fall 1981. The program accepted four students a year into the two-year course. Seated from left to right, the first class included Melissa Church, Huntingdon Area High School, 1981; Mary Huston, Tussey Mountain, 1981; Penny Hall, Southern Huntingdon, 1981; and John Cunningham, Huntingdon Area, 1976. Paul O'Donnell (standing, right) was program coordinator. Funding cuts closed the school in 1985.

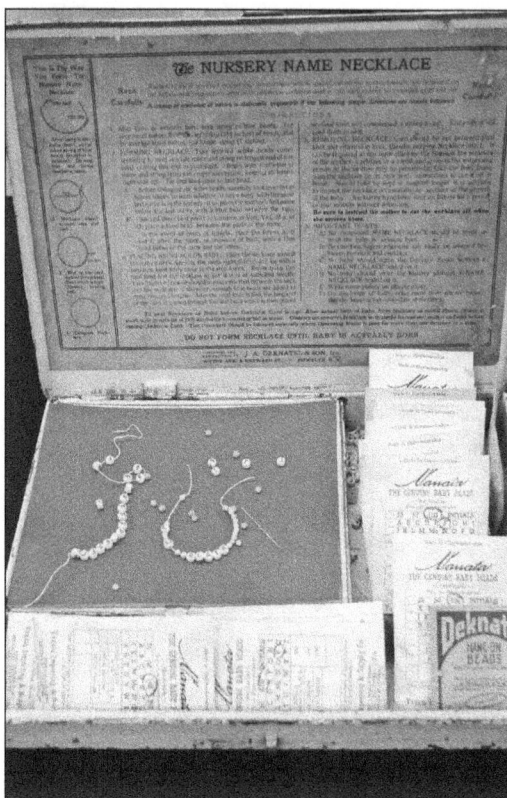

The envelopes in this box hold hundreds of tiny plain blue beads and white beads marked with every letter of the alphabet. These were assembled into little name bracelets for newborn infants to assure that each baby was identified by the mother's last name. The bracelets enabled the nurses to take babies to their mothers at feeding times and ensured that there were no mix-ups at discharge. (Photograph by Linda Cutshall.)

While many mothers carefully preserved the pretty beaded bracelets their babies wore in the hospital, they were probably less likely to save the utilitarian plastic wristbands used later to identify babies. Since 2004, newborns have also been tagged with an electronic ankle bracelet that prevents unauthorized persons from taking a baby from the maternity unit. The auxiliary contributed $36,000 toward installing the $56,000 security system, now required for hospital accreditation.

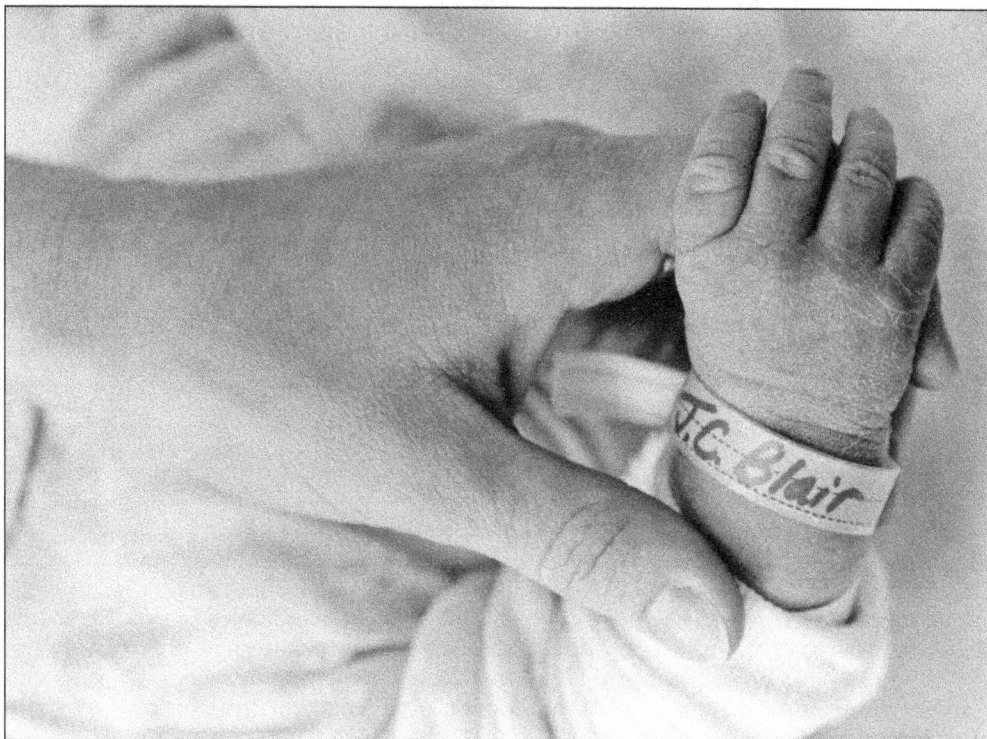

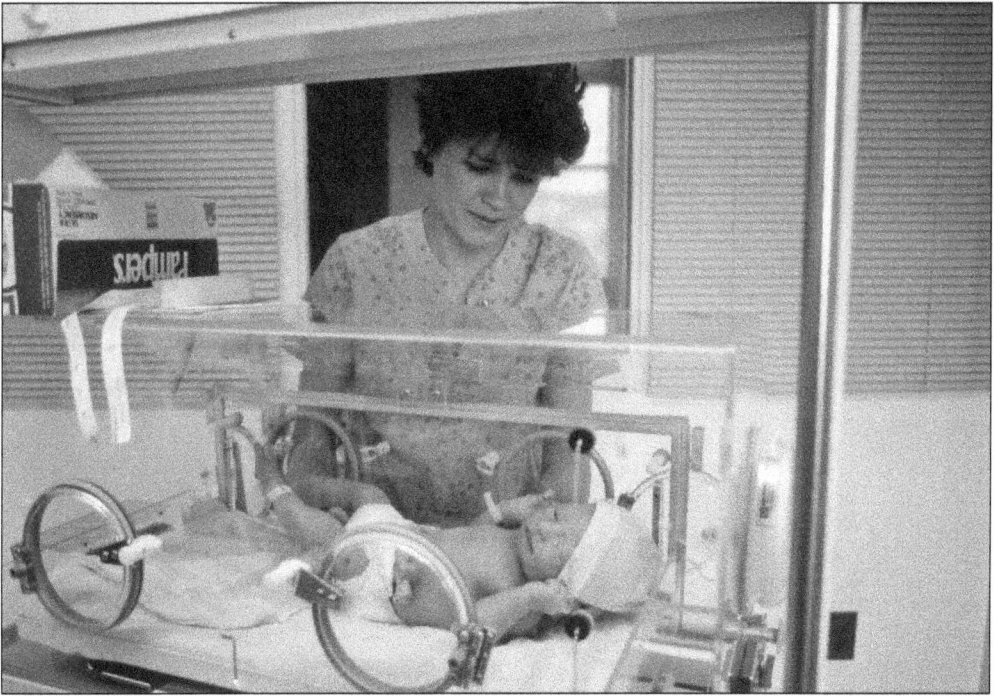

As Marsha Doyle (pictured) knows, caring for premature babies is challenging. On the hospital's 75th anniversary, Mary Alice Ake wrote to say she was born prematurely in Orbisonia in 1916, weighing just 3 pounds. Rushed to J. C. Blair and placed in a bassinet, surrounded by hot water bottles and Mason jars filled with hot water, she survived. "Thanks to you," she wrote, "for helping me to live."

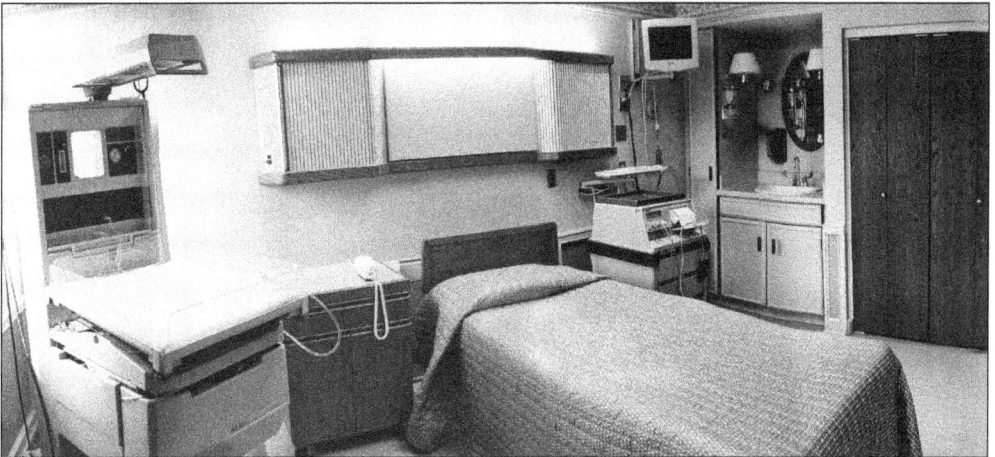

Maternity procedures changed dramatically during Blair Hospital's first century. Today labor and delivery occur in the patient's room, and mother and baby remain there until discharge, in one or two days. A two-week stay for maternity patients was typical through the 1930s, and five to seven days remained standard through the 1950s. Of the 347 babies born at J. C. Blair in 2009, about 90 were delivered by the midwife on staff.

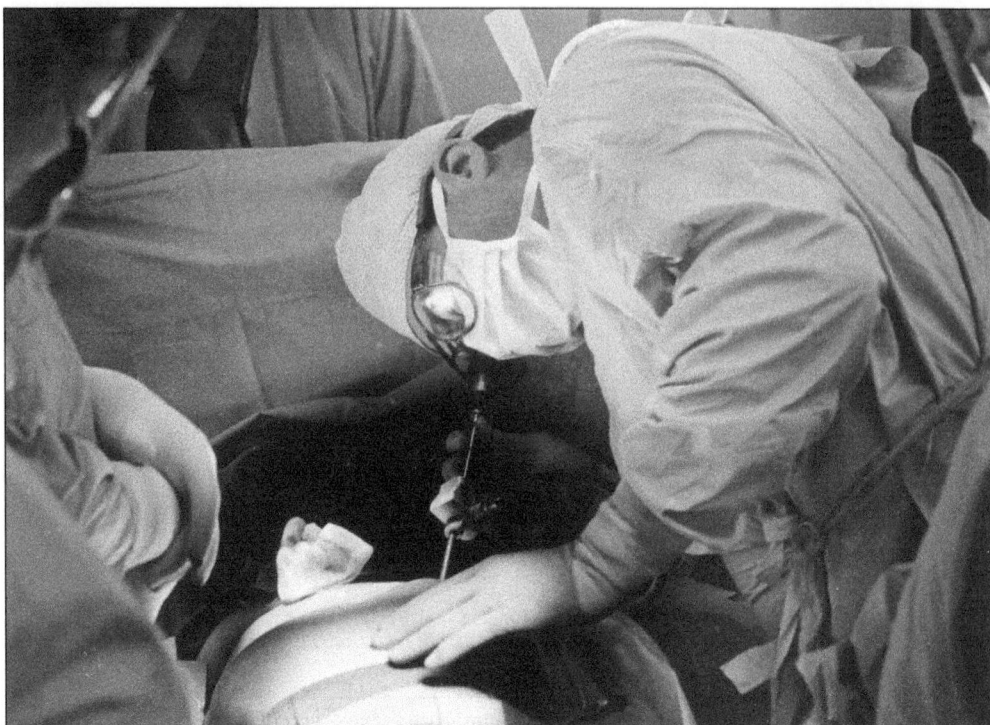

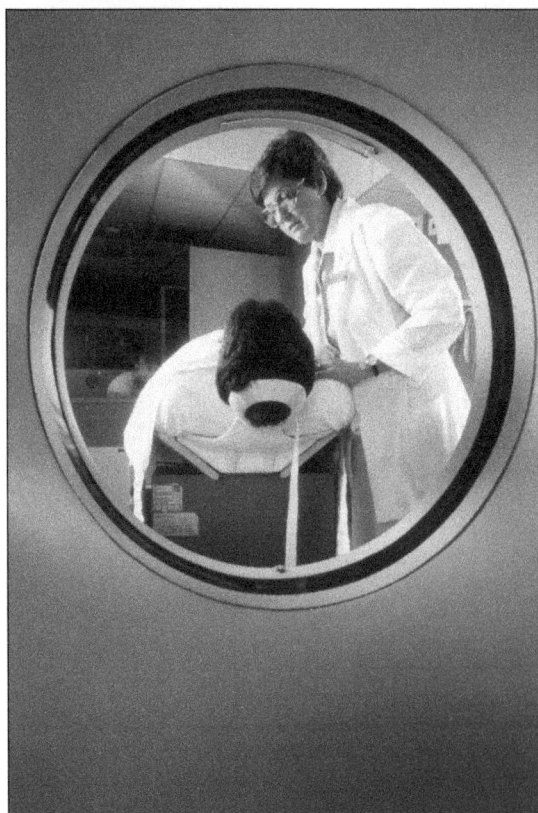

Medical technology, techniques, and procedures have changed and advanced very rapidly in recent years. Here Dr. James L. Hardesty performs minimally invasive laparoscopic surgery, also known as Band-Aid or keyhole surgery. A smaller incision results in faster recovery for the surgical patient and fewer days in a very expensive hospital bed. Many surgeries that used to require a hospital stay are now performed as outpatient procedures.

The development of noninvasive diagnostic imaging technologies such as computerized axial tomography (CAT), mammography, ultrasonography, and magnetic resonance imaging (MRI) have greatly expanded the services provided in Blair's Radiology Department in recent decades. Digital technology has refined the capability of all of these modalities, allowing structures to be identified that are only 1 millimeter in size.

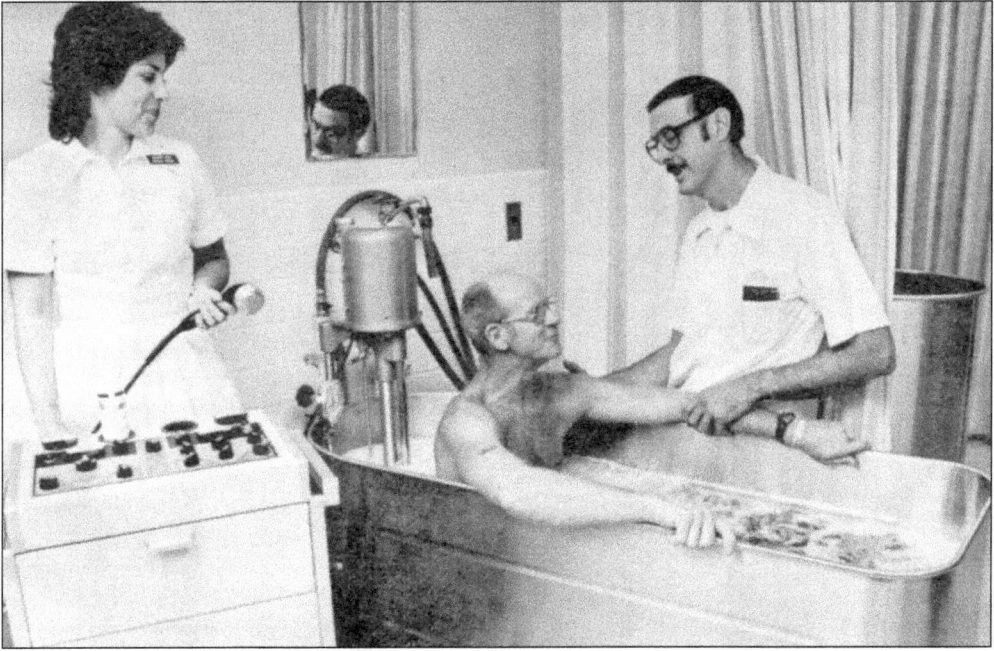

The use of rehabilitative physical therapy in treating postoperative and coronary patients, as well as those with physical limitations or disabilities, has increased dramatically in the years since the hospital hired its first therapist, Ralph Ferrari, in the late 1960s. In this 1980 photograph, Ferrari, then director of the Department of Physical Medicine, and therapy aide Barbara Banks supervise Richard Shearer's treatment in the hydrotherapy whirlpool unit.

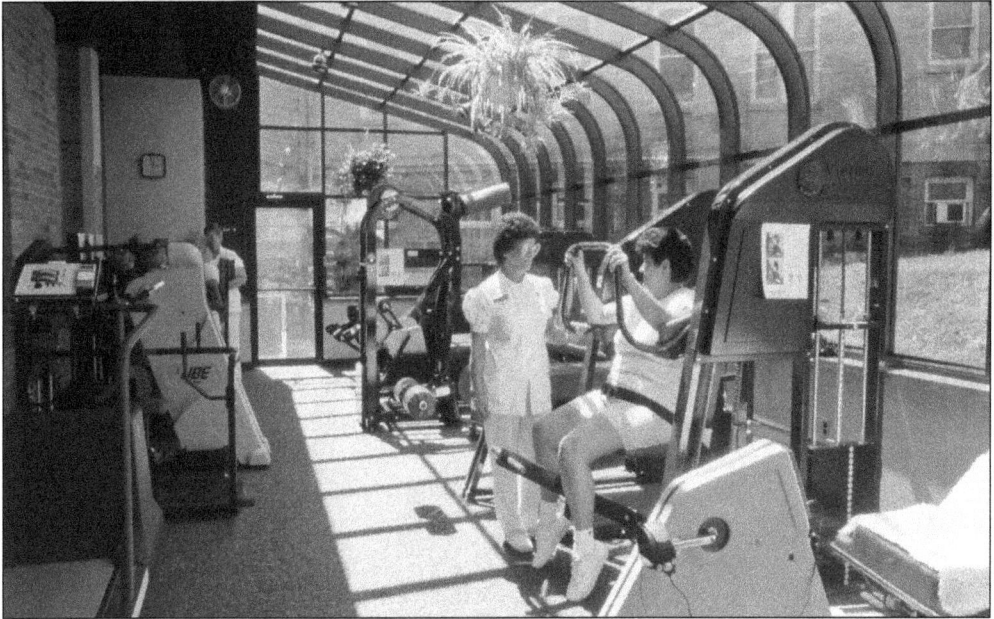

A physical therapy program called Back and Better used this pleasant solarium attached to the hospital's 1972 building. The area was designed by Ralph Ferrari to hold the exercise machines seen here, for the use of patients rehabilitating after surgery or injury—quite different from the more passive uses of the original hospital's solariums.

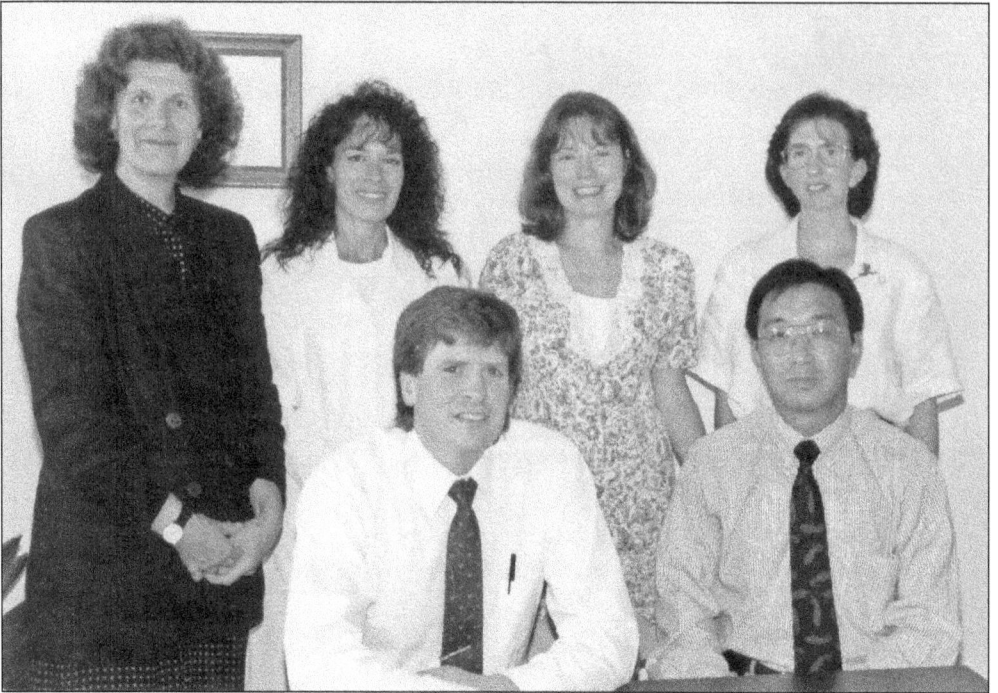

Since 1982, certified nurse midwives (CNM) have offered expectant mothers a new option for pre- and postnatal care and delivery of their babies at J. C. Blair. Standing here are, from left to right, Joann Slattery Condellone, Katherine Curci, Kim Trout, and Sharon McDonough, all certified nurse midwives. Seated in front are consulting obstetricians Dr. Stephen Graham and Dr. Kenneth Lee.

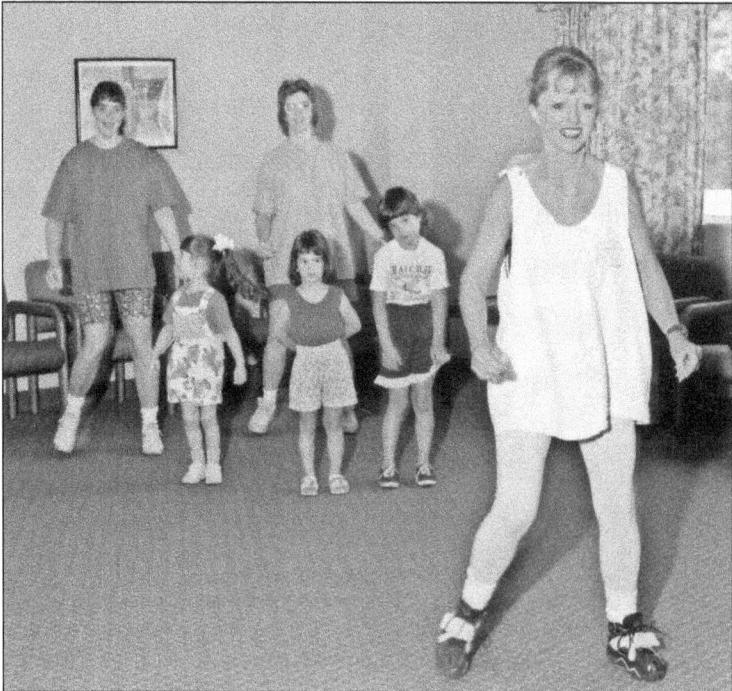

The hospital's Birth and Beyond initiative included an exercise program led by Mary Jane Smith. Birth and Beyond is one of the proactive programs the hospital has offered to promote healthy living. Classes are also offered for expectant parents and for instructing babysitters in caring for the infants and children entrusted to them.

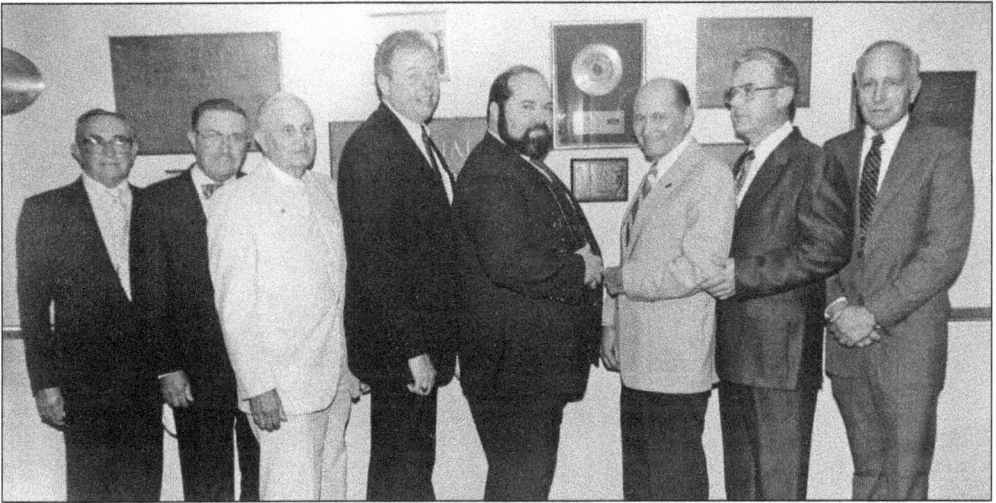

Not every hospital has a gold record in its Hall of History. This one memorializes the first "public" performance of *Mockin' Bird Hill*, by Huntingdon County native and songwriter Vaughn Horton, who sang it for his father, a patient in 1949, and hospital staff who had gathered in his room. Recorded in 1951 by Patti Page and Peter, Paul, and Mary, the song topped the charts for many weeks.

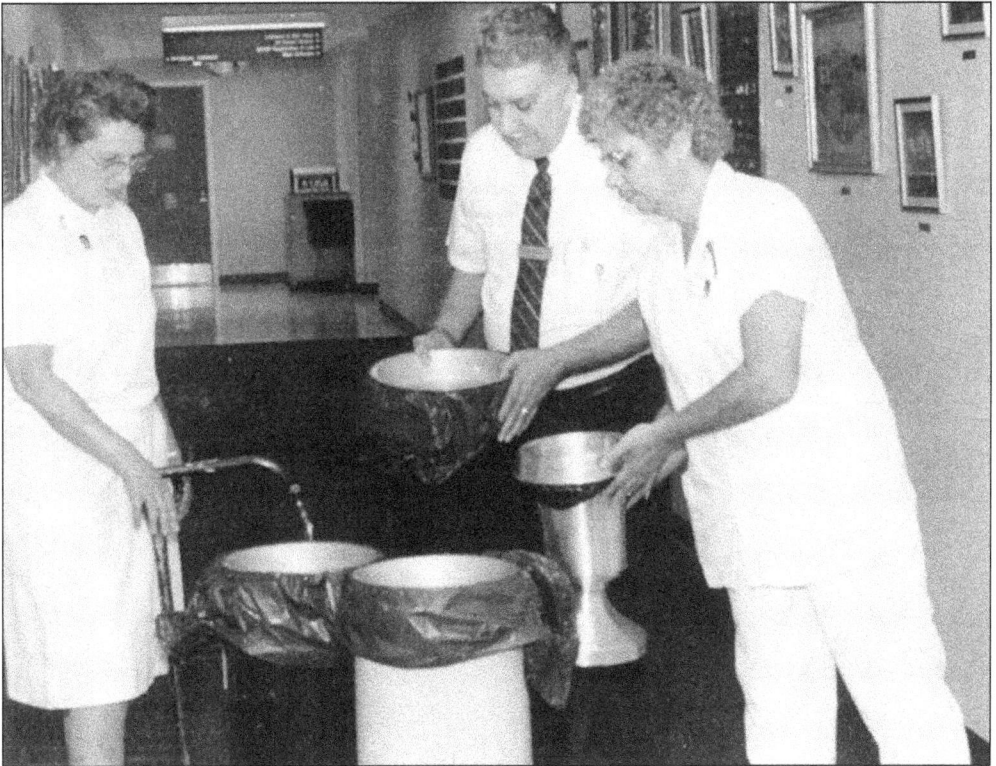

In 1977, the hospital revised its smoking policy to prohibit smoking except in specific areas, but they were numerous and included permitting patients to smoke in their rooms. Not until 1989 was a smoke-free policy adopted. Here, from left to right, Jean Brumbaugh, Morris Nicholson, and Jean Shields remove ashtrays as the ban takes effect.

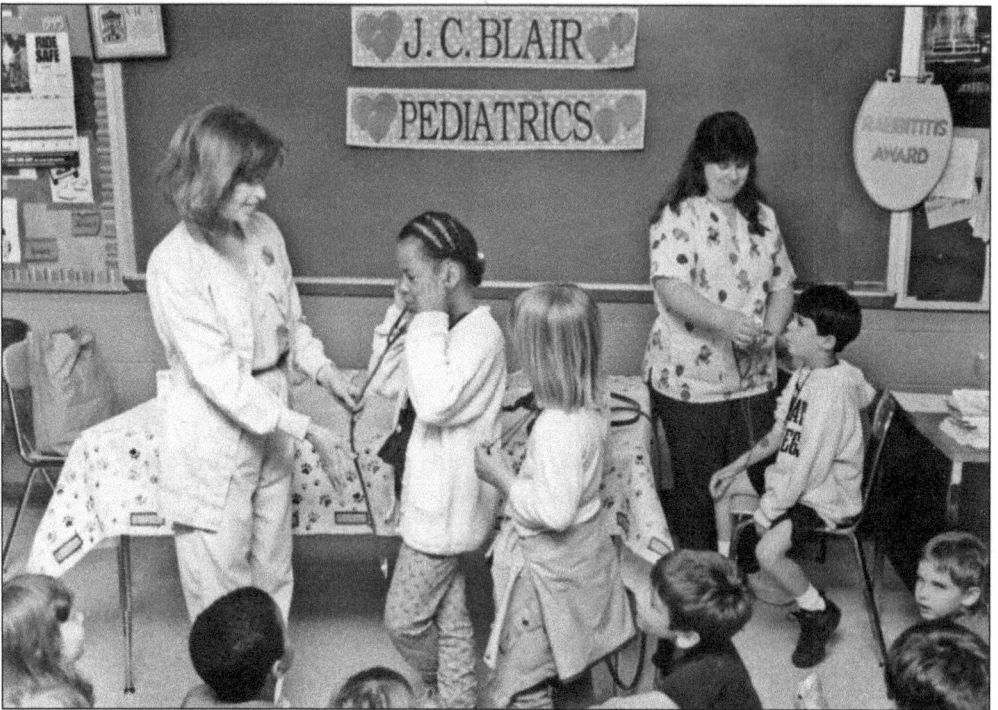

Diane Elliott lets a child try her stethoscope as Kathy Jeffries takes a boy's temperature. They are presenting a program at the annual Children's Health Fair called Preparing for a Hospital Visit, which acquaints children with procedures they would experience if they were hospitalized.

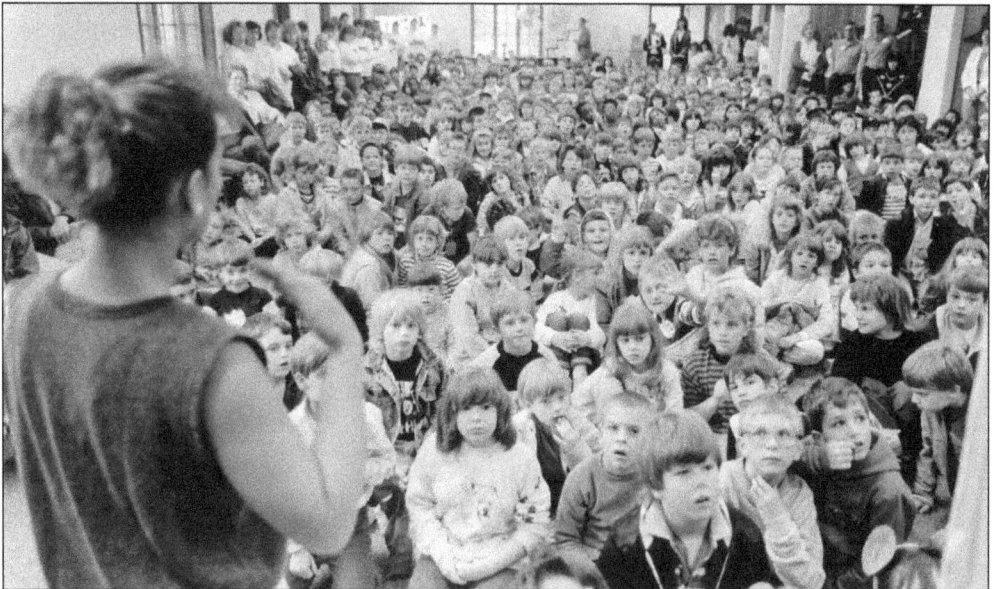

Nearly every third grader in Huntingdon County in 1989 is in this picture. Rain forced the health fair indoors, and this sea of faces was the result. Health fair presentations emphasize good health habits—eating right, caring for your teeth, and exercising, as well as related subjects like bike safety. Such activities go beyond anything the hospital would have seen as within their realm a century ago.

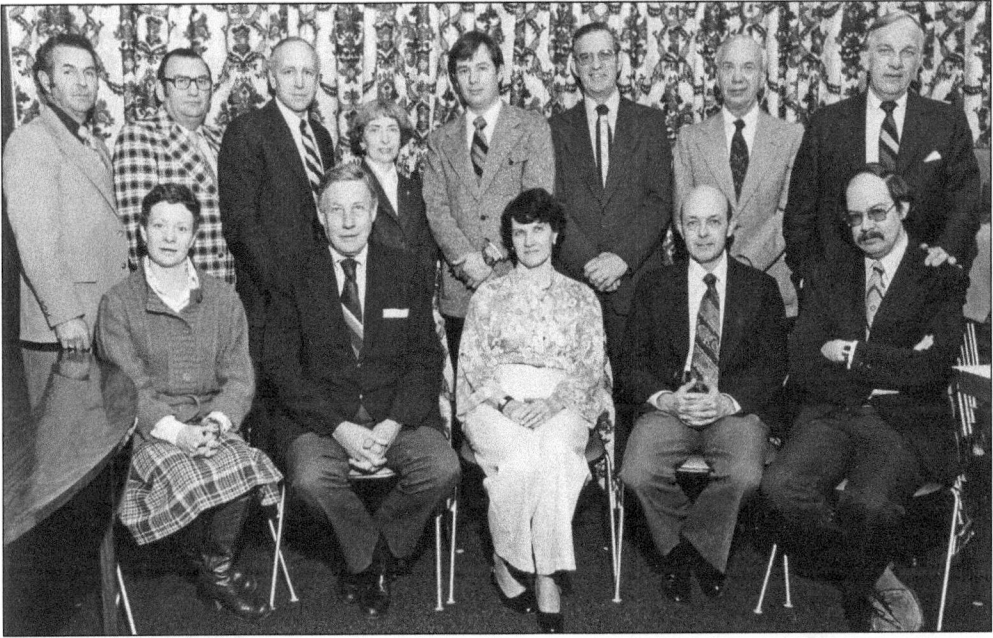

Only men served on the hospital's board of trustees until the 1950s when a seat was designated for the Auxiliary president. In this 1979 photograph, some progress has been made toward gender equity. From left to right are (first row) Pam Thompson, Lynn Corcelius, Nan Hunt, Dr. Thomas Mainzer, and William Russey; (second row) John Pannebaker, Melvin Isett, John B. Kunz, Janet Dore, Philip Thompson, Marshall Showalter, Leonard Fuoss, and Joseph Goodwin.

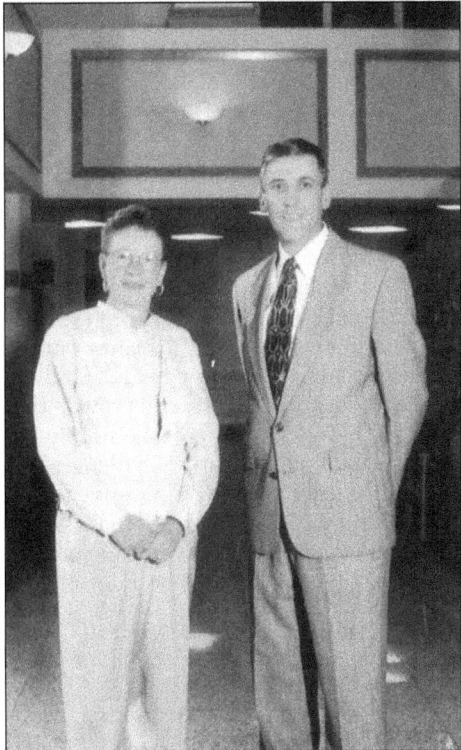

In 1996, Pam Thompson became the first woman to be selected as chairman of J. C. Blair Memorial Hospital's board of directors, as the board has been called since 1988. She brought to the position the commitment evident in her many years of service to the board and the Auxiliary. She is seen here with Richard D'Alberto, then hospital administrator.

125

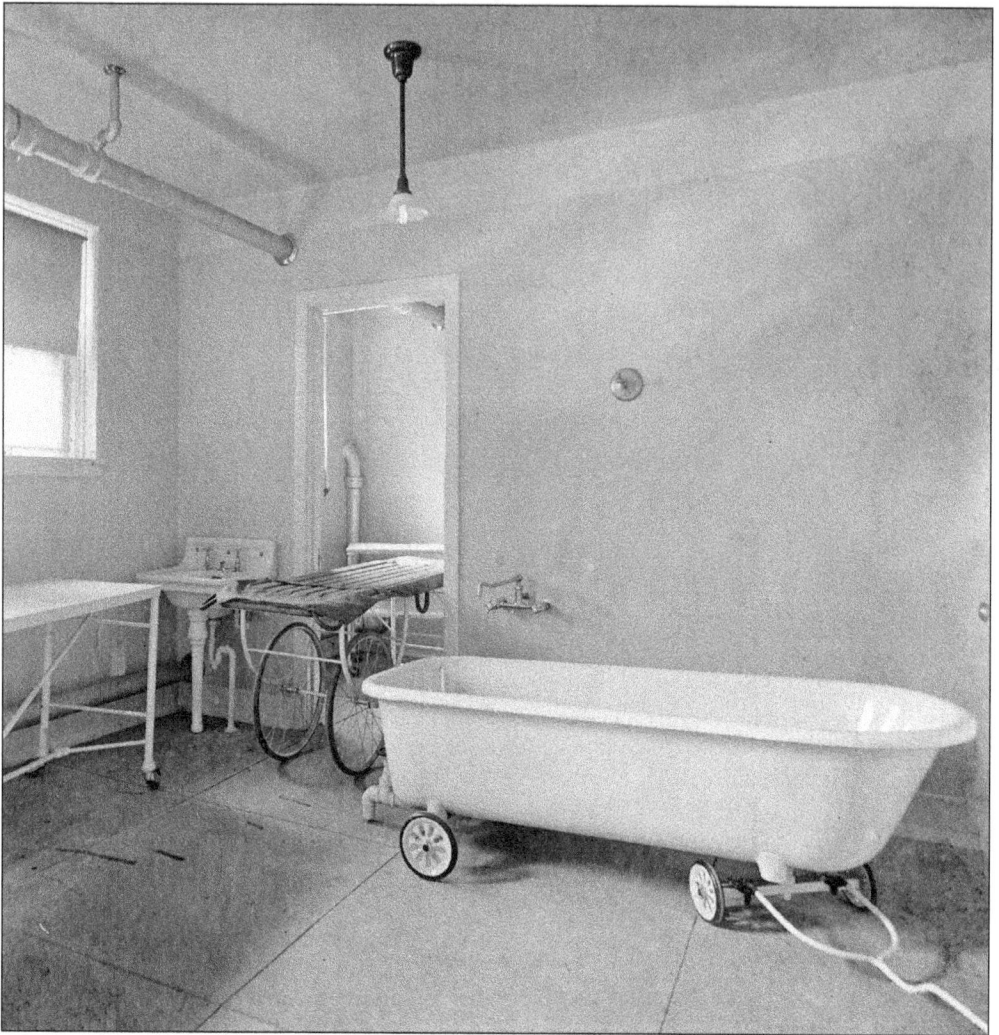

The bathtub on wheels is a favorite vintage hospital image. In the context of the Changing Times chapter, it seems to capture the essence of how times have changed. Yet, in its day, putting wheels on a cast-iron bathtub must have represented innovative thinking. That is a thought worth keeping in mind. Innovation is at the heart of medical science and practice at the beginning of the 21st century, as it has been throughout J. C. Blair Memorial Hospital's first 100 years. Keeping up with the latest advances, in order to provide the community it serves with the best possible medical care, has been a hallmark of the hospital's history. Change has been recognized as a constant. And the difficult and varied challenges that the hospital has faced have been met with resolve and overcome by applying innovative thinking to finding solutions. Putting wheels on a bathtub can stand as a symbol for the hospital's commitment to bringing comfort and care to patients by whatever ingenious means can be found.

AFTERWORD ON SOURCES

The Huntingdon County Historical Society holds a collection of archival documents and photographs important in the history of J. C. Blair Memorial Hospital. These records were essential to the writing of this book. And the society's large photograph collection, including the Blair Shore negative collection, yielded additional important images.

The society's collections also contain a large archive of materials from the J. C. Blair Company, the tablet and stationery company founded by the man to whom the hospital is dedicated. The company's early history was well documented photographically, and a large number of photographs, and the 8-by-10-inch glass negatives from which they were printed, are included in the company archives. The hospital images and negatives are identical in size and were almost certainly by the same photographer.

For almost 75 years, the Huntingdon County Historical Society has been building collections that preserve the history of the county's families, businesses, industries, and communities. It also holds historical county records such as tax assessments and estate inventories. These records are available to the public in the society's historical and genealogical research library.

Considerable information, which advanced the research for this book, was gleaned from the minutes of the hospital auxiliary, from 1913 to 1949, and from scrapbooks that auxiliary members compiled from 1947 to 1997. Many research questions were answered by computer searches of past issues of *The Daily News* and by access to their "morgue," where photographs of and articles about many area doctors were found. Reconstructing a century of hospital history would have been impossible without these records.

Two books, recommended by John B. Kunz and Dr. James E. Savory, illuminated the general context in which the hospital developed: *The Care of Strangers: The Rise of America's Hospital System*, by Charles E. Rosenberg, and *The Social Transformation of American Medicine: The rise of a sovereign profession and the making of a vast industry*, by Paul Starr.

Visit us at
arcadiapublishing.com

www.ingramcontent.com/pod-product-compliance
Lightning Source LLC
Chambersburg PA
CBHW050639110426
42813CB00007B/1854